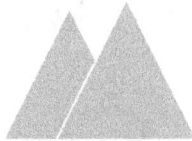

FINDING RE2PITE

When Faith & Fitness
Meet Grace in Suffering

For Jordan

The
sweetest friend
that God ever saw fit
to fearfully and wonderfully make.

TABLE OF CONTENTS

PREFACE
My 2ⁿᵈ Mountain

His love in times past forbids me to think
He'll leave me at last in troubles to sink.
By prayer let me wrestle then He will perform.
With Christ in the vessel, I smile at the storm.
— Olney Hymns

O ur tagline at PrayFit used to be, *"Life is not about the body, but our health is a means of praise."* Some of you may remember that from a decade ago. It's *a little* clunky, somewhat wordy. But despite its lack of rhythm and meter, it's still true. It still holds. Meaning, that any health we have (defined as anywhere between the first and the last heartbeat) is our chance at worship—our one shot at giving glory to His grace.

But the older I get and the longer I spend in the fitness industry, I am growing ever convinced of the complexity of physical stewardship. As if I'm peering into a whirlpool of my own history, and writing, and sin, and illnesses, and breakdowns and breakthroughs, I imagine reaching into the mixture of devotions and pulling that seemingly ancient phrase "means of praise" out of the countless number of words and axioms we've used over the years. Setting it aside, there it is. "Means of praise." Resting my chin in my hands, I ask, *What value do you have in my life and in the lives of my readers, old and new? After all this time, what do you really mean?*

Because in the end, bodily stewardship is just a pathway to worship and service. Bodily stewardship doesn't begin in the gym and end in a flex; rather, it begins and ends in a heart where God is pleased, His image is cherished, and His will is pursued in that process.
Is God pleased?

Is His image cherished?
Is His will pursued in the process?

These are the questions I wish I would have asked myself long before traveling down a thousand roads of health and fitness, especially now, as I navigate illness and suffering. But I'll get into that later.

> *Bodily stewardship doesn't begin in the gym and end in a flex; rather, it begins and ends in a heart where God is pleased, His image is cherished His image is cherished, and His will is pursued in that process.*

Suffice it to say that, as stewards, you and I have been put in charge of something that's not our own, something that God made and gave us to take care of temporarily: these bodies. Of course, that's not anything new or rare to see on this page. It's not exactly the spotted owl. But because of its familiarity, we glaze over that sentence in disregard as if we've just been given the specials menu at our favorite restaurant. But we have to fix our eyes, because, I know in my own life, if the simplest form of bodily stewardship is nothing more than mindful management, I've missed the target muscle completely. If we're not careful, we can *talk* so much about "Faith & Fitness" that we don't do anything—for anyone—with either. Trust me, I know. I've wasted so much of my health on fitness.

I also left too much in the gym; so much that I thought having a good body or just taking care of it meant that I was being a steward. What's more, I even went so far as to use my faith as a platform to show off my body (and vice versa). So silly. I probably would have had my tables overturned in the temple.

> *I've wasted so much of my health on fitness.*

But as I look at the potential emptiness of the old phrase "means of praise," I have to ask myself, after all the books and magazines and blogs and videos, how fit did I have to be to serve people? How healthy is healthy enough to help those without the gift of mobility or those in need of respite? For that matter, how big did my arms have to be in order to *do* something? With the amount of years I spent building them, you'd think the size of my arms actually mattered to the Kingdom.

***

Longtime PrayFit supporter and friend, Roy Gonzalez, said that he ran across a Muscle & Fitness article from 2007 in which I was taking on the reigning Mr. Olympia in a sort of exhibition training session.

It might as well have been yesterday. I drove to Vegas under the impression that the article, "Getting Ready for Mr. O," was to be a story about how the best bodybuilder in the world trains legs as he prepares for the Mr. Olympia contest, and the magazine's fitness editor was going to experience it first-hand; to actually train with him repetition for repetition, set for set. However, I came to find out days later that the writer of the story, Joe Wuebben, was given specific instructions to interview the champ as soon as this editor quit.

He did not get his story.

All those years later, Roy asked me over social media, "What would the 2023 version of Jimmy say to the 2007 version of Jimmy?" My response could not have been more natural. What would I whisper to that Jimmy? Simple. "Don't get under the bar."

But I did. At the end of the training session and photo shoot, when pressed for answers, Mr. Olympia said of me, "He was like a little machine. He would not go away. He was relentless."

Five years later, my eyes had not yet adjusted. After turning out the lights, I stood in pitch blackness. You know the feeling. Though your eyes are wide open, you can't see the end of your nose. So, I did what you would do. I didn't budge. I reasoned that with a new artificial neck and freshly fused spine, the last thing I needed to do was trip and fall. But my wife's eyes had adjusted to the dark. "You're fine, take another step." And there it is. What had to happen for me to move? I needed to have faith that Loretta could see in the dark.

I took so much life out of my body. Sure, I had undetected degeneration and a colon ready to give way, and it certainly wasn't that particular training session with Mr. O that caused my infirmities, but after all these years, look at the resilience of my body. God filled my heart and nerve and sinew with *such* material. I'm a walking miracle. I'm a hard-charging, excitable, stubborn, and tough-to-kill fighter. And I want to serve. I want to play. I want to hike. I want to garden. I want to travel the world to help those in need. I can still do so much more. But I can't pick up my suitcase. That's haunting.

I may be oversimplifying it, but if my body is able to do what it can do now, imagine how capable it would be today had I not been…*so*… foolish. My flesh failed me, yes, but I failed my body too. It had *so much* to give, and I wasted it. God equipped my body for the long haul—for the big battles—and I spent it on little things like fitness. True story. You don't honor God with your body by damaging it under the guise of "bodily stewardship."

> *Honoring God with our bodies has nothing to do with intensity, but has everything to do with intent.*

Silly kingdoms we try to build. Foolish pride. Again, as healthy as I am today, able to do push-ups and planks and stretch and ride my stationary bike, I sometimes imagine how good I would feel and how able I would be to do the *real* work, the kind of work that puts meat on the bones of faith and fitness—the kind of work my heart longs to do for others who don't have the choices I did.

I wish I would have stepped away from that weight. Five hundred and fifty pounds across my back for a few seconds (for who knows how many times over how many years) wasn't worth it. But the best I can do now is to keep walking. No longer in the dark, I want to take another step. And another. By grace, I will fight what would be my natural decline along with the wasting I accelerated, but I will do so in pursuit of real service.

And if you don't read another sentence, please accept this: Honoring God with our bodies has nothing to do with intensity but has everything to do with intent. And based on my record, I had none. Oh, the idea of having strong arms to lift people out of the dirt sounds good on a podcast. It looks great on an Instagram post. But really? I was full of it. Of course I wanted to serve people, but I wanted big arms for the sake of having big arms, and I masked my vain pursuits behind the guise of stewardship.

But I confess, you don't come to that conclusion on the bright, flowery side of the mountain. It doesn't strike you during hilltop moments. You may be *aware* of the truth inside your heart, but you don't admit it up there. No, that kind of wisdom slams you against the wall of the shadowy, quiet side of the mountain; perhaps a second mountain altogether. And when it does, your illusions are exposed as pitiful, pointless mirages, and your swagger trips over your shattered categories.

Sometimes it happens quickly. One day you're taking in a deep inhale, letting the predictable sun warm your face, and the next you're shivering on the cold, dark side of a foreign land you don't recognize. It's a diagnosis that blindsides you, it's the news that binds you, and you wake up miles from reality. And while this instantaneous transport can happen in the blink of an eye, it doesn't always. For some, it's a slow, steady, forced march in a straitjacket toward oblivion.

> *No, that kind of wisdom slams you against the wall of the shadowy, quiet side of the mountain; perhaps a second mountain altogether.*

I'm talking about suffering.

The all shapes and sizes, all makes and models, non-discriminatory, soul-testing forge of suffering. Now, I realize that not all suffering is physical, but all suffering is spiritual.

"Suffering is spiritual warfare," says Pastor Paul Tripp. Why? Because you are not a machine. "If something dysfunctions in a machine, the machine feels no sadness, doesn't worry, doesn't question beliefs, doesn't wish for the life of another machine, and has no concern for what the future holds."

That must be true. It must be war. Because if the gym was my safe castle and fitness my high tower, then suffering scaled the walls of my little kingdom and broke through my pitiful iron gates to—as author C.S. Lewis describes—"plant the flag of truth within the fortress of my rebel soul." If I look across the valley of my life to the first mountain, it looks so small from any distance. Have you ever gone back to visit, say, your elementary school? What you remember as being huge and daunting seems so much smaller, right? That's how my first mountain looks from here. Back then, if the Apostle Paul were to ask me to join him in honoring God with our bodies, I'd try to show him how to lift, but he'd show me who to serve. I'd show him how to eat. He'd show me who to feed. I'd try to show him how to run. He'd show me how to walk.

So small.

But for the Christian in the fitness industry, any exposure to suffering or special needs or invisible illness has the potential to rearrange the furniture of his or her identity. And "exposure" may come through spending time with someone impacted by a disability (with your heart blasted by their joy and purity); or it may come from enduring physical travail yourself, forever altering your expected trajectory. Either way, how you see yourself and, more importantly, how you see God will never be the same. The room will be different. The silly stuff common to the pursuit of health just won't sit right. The fight for process and progress will be accompanied—if not replaced—by purpose and poise.

> *For the Christian in the fitness industry, any exposure to suffering or special needs or invisible illness has the potential to rearrange the furniture of his or her identity.*

Part of life's journey is constant reinvention. A couple of years ago, I returned to my first vocation of hospitality. The symphony of service is a dying art, but as an estate manager, I serve at the pleasure of another. Nothing is about me. I'm a caretaker, the steward of a fortune, merely a custodian. As a leader of fellow servants, my purpose is to point others in the right direction and with the right posture to anticipate what would delight. My job is to pull back the curtain and get out of the way. If I shine, it's only a reflection due to my proximity. I should never be seen. I'm not special, enough, or worthy. My fight is a fight of obscurity.

It's brutal, badass, never-ending, exhausting, and incredibly fulfilling. Radical hospitality is refreshing. All I do is look for feet.

I say all of that because I still rage against the dying of the light, and I battle against my decline, and I have learned to lower my expectations of any kind of fulfillment from achieving physical goals. They mock me because they are so fleeting—a theme I will unpack within the pages of this little book. I strive to be number one, but I am growing increasingly content with second place and, as hospitality has shown me, my place in this world. If my health or illness gets attention and doesn't point others to Christ, I'm not a steward, I'm a thief, stealing something I was never meant to have…the glory.

In the end, fitness was not a friend. Not really. Oh, I tried. We met daily. Thought about him all the time. Did everything he wanted. Anything to keep him around. But then I shook hands with pain and illness—met the real me. Nice to meet you, Jimmy. You're smaller than you look. Weaker than you can imagine. Those are some of your best traits. But it's time to live. Time to die. Suck it up.

And suffering is that friend. Suffering is the friend that introduces a man to himself—the reality that looks you up and down, spits and grins, and then teaches you why you have your next breath. My faith is increasing with every goal I can't reach. It's my diminishing capacity – not my progress – that allows me to see who I really am.

> *Suffering is the friend that introduces a man to himself—the reality that looks you up and down, spits and grins, and then teaches you why you have your next breath.*

Some of you have been with me for ten years. Others of you for almost ten pages. *FINDING RE2PITE* is both the beginning of real purpose and the end of striving. The 2 represents not only a second mountain but our 2 causes of funding mobility and respite. The 2 speaks to the end of mere stewardship and the start of generosity. PrayFit's first mountain, and mine personally, has been conquered. The second mountain, the one of meaning and purpose and vocation… well, it conquered me.

INTRODUCTION
~Lost Tails~
"Perhaps you think too much of your honor, friend."
— Aslan

C onsidered a classic in children's literature, *The Chronicles of Narnia* by C.S. Lewis contains innumerable teaching principles. If you haven't read it—or seen any of the film adaptations—the main character is a lion named Aslan, an alternate version of Jesus in these fantasy tales.

Wiping away tears at the end of each film, my wife Loretta and I agree that if we could hug Aslan, we'd do so and never let go. We'd follow him everywhere, never letting him out of our sight. If the most gentle and powerful being of all time were our closest friend and at our side day and night, we'd have the courage to talk about God with anyone, anywhere, anytime. We'd forgive sooner and help more—and don't get us started on how much less we'd worry. And of course, I wonder what Aslan would say about the body, how we handle our health and illness. Actually, I think C.S. Lewis gives us an idea in one incredible scene.

Picture Aslan talking to Reepicheep, a brave, sword-fighting mouse who has lost his tail in a great battle. While Aslan assures and tries to encourage Reepicheep by telling him the shortened tail becomes him well, Reepicheep *dramatically* offers his sword to Aslan, saying that because of his deformity he must resign from duty. Cue the drama. Extending his sword, bending the knee, and bowing his head:

"All the same, great King. I regret that I must withdraw, for a tail is the *honor and glory* of a mouse," Reepicheep says.

"Perhaps you think too much of *your honor*, friend," Aslan replies.

When I lost my "fitness"—*my* honor and glory—I thought I was done. Like Reepicheep, I thought too much of myself, as if physical stewardship and helping others through their journeys had anything to do with the survival of my own body. But that's the unenjoyable blessing of suffering. Suffering is honest.

Suffering shatters our categories and crushes our suppositions. Suffering whispers in your ear the truth, that life's pleasures will flatter us as they arrive and mock us as they leave. And that moment will hurt all the more if that pleasure is our treasure. Which of course, it was to me. I won't sugarcoat it. The suffering I'm talking about isn't watered down. I'm not talking about the kind of suffering that's accompanied by "enjoyable" pain; in my old training days, the temporary, tough, voluntary, and *enjoyable* pain told me I would get to my goals.

> *Suffering shatters our categories and crushes our suppositions.*

No, the suffering I'm talking about is the same kind many of you are going through. And I want to be extremely sensitive here; I don't say or type the word "suffering" easily. When I first met Joni Eareckson Tada and served under her leadership for a time, and as I've watched her live her life, the concept of suffering took on new meaning. It became sacred, almost to the point that I questioned my ability to write on the subject. So I tread very carefully. You'll learn more about Joni in the coming pages, but suffice it to say that compared to her, I have never really suffered. But I will say that in my journey and study, I've come to learn that there are varying degrees of suffering—down to the kind that's accompanied by a pain you never saw coming. A pain you don't know if you can endure because you don't know if it will ever end. The kind of pain that's disorienting because you can't remember what it felt like *not* to hurt. The kind of pain that's accompanied by excruciating, debilitating, humiliating misery.

"Suffering drags you deeper into yourself," says David Brooks. "It smashes you through a floor you thought was the bottom floor of your soul, revealing a cavity below, and then it smashes through that floor, revealing another cavity, and so on and so on. The person in pain descends to unknown ground. Suffering opens up ancient places that have been hidden. When people are thrust down into these deeper zones, thrust into lonely self-scrutiny, they are forced to confront the fact that they can't determine what goes on there. It shatters the illusion of self-mastery. It teaches gratitude. We realize how undeserving we are."

Far be it from me to try to unpack and measure the heights and depths of suffering with any measure of success. Again, in my journey, I lean on heroes of the faith like Joni, Dr. Charles Spurgeon, Paul Tripp, David Brooks, Tim Challies, Max Lucado, and, of course, Tim Keller to carry me to the throne of grace on the subject. But for this corner of the world, and from my limited perspective, I can tell you that suffering impacts the physical, emotional, and relational cores of our being. Regardless of the source and kind of travail you or I have, it reaches the depths and heights of everything we're made of (until we find out what we're made of).

In order to arrive there, I've structured this project into three main sections. But let me first say, *FINDING RE2PITE* is *not* a roadmap of health or suffering. I would know. Throughout my career, I've written hundreds of articles and a nice handful of books that contained specific instructions on the what, why, and how of achieving a particular goal. But *FINDING RE2PITE* is not that kind of book. It's actually more of a diary, a description of the road with less focus on how to cross it. Nobody knows exactly how to do that.

But imagine, if you will, an uninvited stranger knocks on your door. Before you can answer, he opens the door with his own key, steps inside, hands you his coat, puts his luggage in the master bedroom, heads to the kitchen and makes himself a sandwich. Before you know it, he's rearranging the furniture and sitting in your chair.

"Can I help you?"

"Nope, I'm good. But I'm here to let you know that your life will never be the same. All those dreams? Gone. Those passions? Goals? Professional trajectory? History. And your body? Well, it won't ever function the same again. Get ready for a pain you're not sure will ever go away, combined with a nagging doubt in your head that you can actually withstand it. Anxiety, insomnia, depression…all in play. Your joy will be at risk. Your relationships could suffer. Your self-worth will be subject to whether or not you're anchored to something far more stable than grit or guts or discipline, which, by what I know of you, is in question despite your social media feed. On this side of heaven, my presence in your life has the potential to feel like the worst parts of the Bible. And it's not a dream."

Absurd? Maybe. But that's how suffering enters your life. Your identity and the life patterns and the decisions you make, and the common denominators of your life that you thought would be there for the long haul, are removed without your consent; to say nothing about the pain that comes with it. Nigerian writer Chinua Achebe once said, "When suffering knocks at your door and you say there is no seat for him, he tells you not to worry because he has brought his own."

But the story isn't over. Here's another impossible twist to what you thought was fiction. What happens when the stranger—over time—becomes a sort of *friend*? Someone you never knew (or wanted) that barges into your life and over time, and by the grace of God, helps you become someone you couldn't be otherwise. By grace, he has helped you become more compassionate, humble, loving, empathetic, and forgiving.

Do you wish he had never come into your life? Yes and no. But he helps you see how some things in life were just too important to you. He helped rearrange your thoughts and your wills and even your skills at navigating life, to the point that you wonder how far off course you were before you met. Eventually, you both decide that while life didn't turn out the way you had planned, there really are places to go and people to meet.

And just as you open the door to embark upon a new life, you call for him to join you. And while he doesn't answer, somehow you know he's coming with you. You step outside and walk to the curb and look back at a house, or a gym, or a job, or a body that once meant so much to you. In that moment, everything seems *less*. Less pressing. Less fulfilling. Less dramatic. It's like your eyes have adjusted for the first time and you realize that whatever it is you're going to do, or wherever you're going, won't be as difficult or as confusing.

Suffering broke your spirit. Suffering taught you the meaning of smallness, dependence, and weakness and shaped your humility. Suffering stopped you from navel gazing, raised your chin and your line of sight, and eventually your horizon. Suffering made things smaller, especially you. And now, it's time to go. Turns out, God never needed your body.

Breaks, Shapes, Sends

And with that mental picture, I've sectioned the book into three main themes. And while some chapters could easily be placed into multiple sections, they are as such:

> Suffering taught you the meaning of smallness, dependence, and weakness and shaped your humility.

Section One: Suffering breaks us.
Section Two: Suffering shapes us.
And finally, section three: Suffering sends us.

Pretty simple. It's just...you don't come to each simply. Each section—like a piece of artwork or a song or a mission or a vocation—can take a lifetime to appreciate. You may be reading this page and know exactly where you fall, but if you don't know, you may in the end.

Suffering...
Breaks us. Down to size.
Shapes us. Into someone you don't recognize (or so you thought).
Sends us. To serve people and see places and fill spaces you never would have otherwise.

And I think that's a perfect way to begin this little book, a book written for...

The fitness enthusiast. For the person who has a passion for fitness, but who also wants to wrap their hard-charging heart around the purpose and idea of real suffering.

The trainer. For the person who teaches others how to be fit, or how to lose some weight, or improve their strength, flexibility, and endurance, all while not knowing their client may have disorienting pain (or perhaps they *are* aware). But they want to have a fresh, godly perspective on bodily stewardship—and a sensitivity for—their client's possible travail. **The dietitian**. For the person who knows the value of healthy nutrition and teaches others how to manage macronutrients, while also wanting to know the Biblical perspective of pain and chronic illness for both themselves and their clients.

The gym owner. For he or she who *employs* those with invisible chronic pain. It's for the gym owner who *serves* guests and customers with invisible chronic pain. It's for the gym owner who *has* invisible chronic pain.

It's for **the caregiver, family member, or friend** who needs to know a stitch of the "why" and the "what" of suffering and pain, and how they can rest in the sovereignty of God for their own sanity while providing genuine care and comfort to those they love.

This book is for **the healthy and strong**; for the one who may never have battled with anything or been a blip on the radar of pain or setbacks. It's for those that still believe you always get what you work for; that health is earned, and strength and ability are measures of how much you "want" it.

And this book is for **the sick, the hurting, the pain-stricken, and the constant sufferer.** For those who have been invaded. For the one who wants to scratch the surface on the Biblical view of suffering and gain a few thoughts and perspectives from those who have gone through (or are living through) the travail of pain. If you suffer or know someone who does, I wrote this book for you.

Friends, someday we'll have eternal bodies. My current aches, pains, and restrictions are clear and present reminders of that hope. One day we'll double over, not in pain, but in praise. One day, our knees won't crackle and our bones won't break. No more back problems or stomach aches. No more cancer, heart disease, diabetes, or sore throats. Someday.

Until then, I, like you, will try to take care of my body, trusting God, with the results as His gifts and my limits just the same. Doing both takes grace.

May this work be a source of comfort for the hurting and struggling, and a source of inspiration and motivation for those who see today—maybe for the first time—as a day to make bodily stewardship a means of praise. This broken and groaning body carries the soul, so may how we treat it be a small, silent, humble way of showing respect for that honor.

May we deal with our debilitating aches and our private pain with an uncommon grace, and help others do the same. May our abilities and our disabilities, our personal records and our medical records, carry a message to the world that, although we grow weary, we are the Body. Lost tails and all.

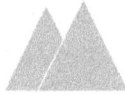

SECTION ONE
Suffering Breaks Us

What if a master sculptor was working on a piece of granite, and the granite objected to the many chips falling to the floor. The granite feels that the Master has gone too far. That kind of thinking would be incomprehensible. So be assured the Master Craftsman knows exactly what He's doing. His primary intention is for you to "go on unto perfection" (Heb 6:1). And he'll stop short of nothing to accomplish this end. He'll interrupt your life without asking your permission.

— A.W. Tozer

~This Is Gonna Hurt~
God had one Son on earth without sin, but never one without suffering.
— Augustine

The white chairs outside the Garden Tomb in Israel were warm from the sun. The tour was almost over, and the next day would be our last in Jerusalem. When our Pastor, Shawn Thornton, began reading about those six hours on Good Friday, it was as if I had felt my skin for the first time. I was doing business with God.

Stooping inside that ancient tomb…
I was Thomas seeing scars.
I was a flat-footed Peter looking at my feet on the waves.
I was the woman at the well.
I was both the mocking criminal and the soon-to-be saint.
I was Bartimaeus after receiving his sight, and the rich young ruler afraid to part with his toys.
I was an arrogant Saul blinded by grace.
I was the shouting leper diving at Jesus' feet.

And I was Jacob, limping through the streets in the early morning dawn. Storefronts are opening for business while owners sweep the front porches. Roosters are greeting the day, dogs scamper away from food left in the streets, and neighbors are sipping their Hebrews java.
And here comes Jacob. Dragging one leg as a testimony to his time with God…

Genesis Chapter 32:22-31
[22] *During the night Jacob got up and took his two wives, his two servant wives, and his eleven sons and crossed the Jabbok River with them.* [23] *After taking them to the other side, he sent over all his possessions.*
[24] *This left Jacob all alone in the camp, and a man came and wrestled with him until the dawn began to break.* [25] *When the man saw that he would not win the match, he touched Jacob's hip and wrenched it out of its socket.* [26] *Then the man said, "Let me go, for the dawn is breaking!" But Jacob said, "I will not let you go unless you bless me."*
[27] *"What is your name?" the man asked.*

He replied, "Jacob."

²⁸ "Your name will no longer be Jacob," the man told him. "From now on you will be called Israel, because you have fought with God and with men and have won."

²⁹ "Please tell me your name," Jacob said.

"Why do you want to know my name?" the man replied. Then he blessed Jacob there.

³⁰ Jacob named the place Peniel (which means "face of God"), for he said, "I have seen God face to face, yet my life has been spared." ³¹ The sun was rising as Jacob left Peniel, and he was limping because of the injury to his hip.

Jacob held on. Just wouldn't let go. Not until he got his blessing. Jacob went through something that forever changed how he related to God. The Lord weakened him physically to strengthen him spiritually. Expecting the worst from his brother Esau, Jacob not only prepared practically (sending Esau gifts ahead of his arrival) but he talked to God. *A lot.* Then one night the Bible says he wrestled with a mysterious man. As the fight continued, the man touched and dislocated Jacob's hip. And that was enough to convince Jacob that this was no ordinary man, but in fact he saw God (v.30). So he held on, refusing to let go until he received his blessing.

Battle-tested and blessed, Jacob had two new things: a limp and a name.

The limp is significant to me personally because Jacob knew that in his new physical state, he would never be able to defend himself against Esau. He had to rely on God, and God alone, to fight his battles. Not sure about you, but I know more than ever that I'm weaker than I think. Oh, I know that goes against what the world boasts, but like Jacob, even Paul understood that we rely more on God when we embrace our smallness.

What did Paul say? "I am content in my weakness...for when I'm weak, I'm strong." I really didn't understand that verse until I was humbled to the dirt. But gracefully, I feel stronger in my weakness than I ever felt in my strength.

And as far as Jacob's new name, well, he went from "heel

catcher, *Jacob*" to "he who struggles with God, *Israel*." Indeed, there's no better way to walk through life than with a limp that says you've been with God.

Alistair Begg says that the thing we fear the most could be exactly what God uses to bless us. That could be in unfamiliar terms or territory, or a removal of support systems, but in mysterious ways, God will lead us into His presence to get our attention.

And in this case, God took Jacob alone to work out the process in his life. The moment was as painful as it was permanent. But that's where he blessed him. Notice that before he blessed Jacob, he weakened him. (v.25) "The reason we have so little of the blessing," says Begg, "is because we are unprepared for the crippling...in this success-oriented society where we feel the blessed are only the healthy and wealthy."

> *Indeed, there's no better way to walk through life than with a limp that says you've been with God.*

Joni Eareckson Tada, founder and CEO of Joni & Friends International Disability Center, agrees. "Jacob's personal encounter with God made all the difference and forever changed him," says Joni. "He could now be used. When Jacob returned home, he was a broken man. He had suffered greatly, much of it the result of his own sin. But in the end, Jacob serves as one of the most dramatic Biblical pictures of how brokenness and suffering can radically transform an individual's character and life's trajectory when touched by the power of God."

God breaks him to bless him. Jacob walks away blessed but weaker; not your typical "faith & fitness" slogan. But notice that Jacob says he will not let him go. Why? He knew that the most important thing was to be blessed by God. His greatest need, like ours, is to be blessed by God, blessed to have a passion for God and to hunger and thirst for His Word. But we cling to the wrong things. I know I do. It's so hard to let go of the wrong things in order to hold tight to what's right. Sometimes we need God to help us rip them from our fingers.

A.W. Tozer describes it like this: "There is within the human heart a tough fibrous root of fallen life whose nature is to possess, always to possess. It covets "things" with a deep and fierce passion. The roots of our hearts have grown down into things, and we dare not pull up one rootlet lest we die. But the ancient curse will not go out painlessly. He must be torn out of our heart like a plant from the soil. He must be expelled from our soil by violence."

Jacob had a testing place with God, where he was found both crippled by and clinging to God. Have you faced a testing point? "If we are set upon the pursuit of God," says Tozer, "He will sooner or later bring us to the testing place, and we may never know when we are there. At that testing place there will be no dozen possible choices for us—just one, and an alternative—but our whole future will be conditioned by the choice we make."

And as Jacob held on to God, the test went the way many wrestling matches go: When you're down on the mat, and the wrestler has his grip on you—the grip that has made you powerless—fighting isn't the way out of his grasp. Surrender is.

Cutting to the chase, if our pursuit of fitness or our battle with chronic pain and illness isn't leading us to surrender our lives toward a deeper relationship with God, then that ache—*the deepening root*—that buries itself within our fibers and nourishes our desire (for either strong bodies or the healing of our pain) needs to be uprooted by force. And it's not painless. It doesn't go away easily. It doesn't lie down in obedience.

But it's when we stop fighting, stop comparing, stop striving, and stop masking that we overcome the enemy. It's when we tap out—even if it means being in worse physical shape or in the midst of chronic pain and unbearable loss—that we gain all things. It's when we *surrender* that "ours is the Kingdom of Heaven." It's in those moments of limp weakness, when stubborn rock softens, that we begin to embrace the kind of strength that God is wanting us to pursue.

But we have this treasure in jars of clay,
to show that the surpassing power belongs to God and not to us...
— 2 Corinthians 4:7

We're dust and God knows it, and He has compassion. "God breathed on clay and it became a man. God breathes on man and he becomes clay," says Tozer. The apostle Paul himself said that we have this treasure inside these bodies, these jars of clay, to show that the power belongs to God and not to us. Now, compare what Paul said to something I read on a picture quote recently, where someone boastfully warns, "Before you judge me, step into my shoes and walk the life I'm living, and if you get as far as I am, just maybe you'll see how strong I really am."

I admit, I'd love to hear Paul's graceful response to such a charade, because if the most influential man this side of Christ knew anything, he knew where his power and strength came from and where they didn't. Can you imagine Paul talking about how strong he is? And yet, you and I battle with pride about it.

See, to Paul, surviving the shipwreck or sustaining the beatings wasn't so much death-defying as much as it was life-revealing. Suffering was bringing about perseverance and purpose in his life.

And to think, you're a jar of clay. So am I. A malleable, bendable, fillable, and spillable jar of clay. I know some days we feel more like a piñata than a Godly jar of clay, but if you hit a piñata hard enough, what happens? Others get the treasure inside. And that's what I get from Paul. He bled Jesus. He bled the treasure.

This book is designed to help you let go of all levels of "self" until you're broken and spilled out. It's complex, right? Especially among hard chargers and fighters, the sick and healthy alike. In fact, you may be soldiering through illness, or you may be strolling through perfect wellness, but the ground is level. Please hold on. This book is written in both languages.

With Mighty Blows

By the time Pastor Shawn got to the part about the stone being rolled away from the Garden Tomb, I had become a malleable mess. My frail little body was merely a few feet away from where Jesus made it well with my soul. And when I took communion in that Garden, Jesus wrote a note in the dirt and I became clay.

Dear friends, as we progress through this book, let's invite others to step into our shoes and live the lives we're living. And when they get as far as we've gone, maybe—*just maybe*—they'll get to see exactly just how strong *we're not*. For us to be of any use to God, something has to break. Right now, you may be in suffering's grip with no way out. It's not gonna be painless. It's going to hurt. But to get out, just hang on and surrender.

When God wants
to drill a man
And thrill a man
And skill a man,
When God wants to mold a man
To play the noblest part;

When He yearns with all His heart
To create so great and bold a man
That all the world shall be amazed,
Watch His methods, watch His ways!

How He ruthlessly perfects
Whom He royally elects!
How He hammers him and hurts him,
And with mighty blows converts him.
Into trial shapes of clay which
Only God understands;
While his tortured heart is crying
And he lifts beseeching hands!

How He bends but never breaks
When his good He undertakes;
How He uses whom He chooses,
And which every purpose fuses him;
By every act induces him
To try His splendor out...
God knows what He's about.

— Anonymous

~Dirt for a Mirror~

When you become consumed by God's call on your life, everything will take on new meaning and significance. You will begin to see every facet of your life – including your pain – as a means through which God can work to bring others to Himself.
— Charles Stanley

I'd say he honored God with his body. He baptized almost 15,000 members, maintained a weekly attendance of 6,000 people, and spawned 66 para-church ministries, including two orphanages and a theological college. By 1892, he had published more words in the English language than any other Christian in history. Without the aid of television, radio, or the internet, he proclaimed the gospel of Jesus Christ to an estimated 10 million people in his lifetime. And he did it sick.

Indeed, Dr. Charles Spurgeon had his share of deep, painful physical needs. So painful in fact, that in 1886 he said, "When I am suffering very greatly from gout, if anybody walks heavily and noisily across the room, it gives me pain." In his autobiography he wrote, "I thought a cobra had bitten me and filled my veins with poison. I think it would have been less painful to have been burned alive at the stake than to have passed through those horrors and depressions of spirit."

As if Spurgeon were talking directly to me from centuries ago, he writes, "O dear friend, when thy grief presses thee to the very dust, worship there! If that spot has come to be thy Gethsemane, then present there thy 'strong crying and tears' unto thy God. Turn the vessel upside down, and let every drop run out; but let it be before the Lord. When you are bowed down beneath a heavy burden of sorrow, then take to worshipping..." (Spurgeon; from the Sermon *Job's Resignation*)

It's no wonder Spurgeon was able to connect with his audience. He understood. And it's no wonder he said, "The greatest earthly blessing that God can give to any of us is health, with the exception of sickness." But from experience, when it comes to pain, weakness, smallness, frailty, and neediness, the fit and fiddle mock it. The strong and independent vilify it. But the blind, the lame, the beggars, the sick, the suffering, and the souls upon the coals, they kiss it. Because when strivings cease and the muscle fades and it only hurts to breathe, that's when the dirt becomes the mirror. When you're staring into the sand and you wonder if this is how it ends, or if this is as good as it will ever be, or where it all went. Yeah, that's when you kiss it.

I remember lying in my bathtub. A year removed from my neck replacement surgery and two from my back reconstruction, I was dealing with something far more severe. Most of you know that I had a colon infirmity where a spasm prevented me from being able to function normally, and the two-year daily war with pain was unbearable. For months leading up to that risky surgery—in my bathtub with water full of blood and waste—I'd cry, I'd worry, I'd get angry, I'd apologize to my body, I'd question. Until one day, I resigned. Those that have my latest book recall my journal entry:

> *Because when strivings cease and the muscle fades and it only hurts to breathe, that's when the dirt becomes the mirror.*

I never predicted such weeks like this.
If I ever get up...if I ever hope and rise and stand...if I ever smile, truly smile and speak and write and encourage, make no mistake, it won't be because I kept fighting. It won't be because of my inner man, my deep faith or some gut-summoned passion of belief. No, I have none of that. If I ever get better, it will only be by the mercy and unbelievable, inconceivable grace of my dear God.

Now, this will sting, but to a "faith & fitness" industry—filled with its meadow maidens striking a pose under the guise of faith while verse-splattered tank tops with their easily devised metaphors fill your social media feed—Dr. Charles Spurgeon has plenty to teach us. Some of you reading this sentence could likely add to this little chapter's content, I'm sure, because your feet still throb from the coals of pain and illness. But what in life ever drops you to your knees? What makes your knees buckle? Is it in praise and gratefulness of high achievement? It should be, but for me, no. I usually collapse in hardship, sin, chronic illness, and suffering. I fold like a chair when I find the end of me and realize I am completely useless.

Dwayne "The Rock" Johnson says (smoldering), "It's not enough to be hungry. You have to starve for greatness." Don't get me wrong, I like Dwayne. Got to hang way back in the day. Super nice guy, hard-working, and I'm nobody to argue with him. But that "starve for greatness" mentality will leave you gasping and flopping around like a fish on a hot sidewalk. Yup. Funny, the world says, "starve for greatness," but the Bible says to feed people. Ironic.

Anyway, when I rolled into L.A. nearly 20 years ago to be the fitness director at Muscle & Fitness magazine, everything worked—body cranking, books flying. Starving for greatness and eating like a machine. I wasn't praying for daily bread. I have never been that hungry (or generous) that I prayed for daily bread and meant it. I was too busy meal-prepping. There wasn't anything I couldn't conquer "by faith." But that's hogwash. Silly kingdoms we build. Fast-forward and you'll find what can only be described as broken, gutted, and humbled. But that's just me. The same goes for the old Weider building. The worldwide M&F headquarters has long been sold and - at the time of this paragraph - is being demolished.

I used to strut down those halls, jeans filled out, full of power and strength, thinking that I earned my body while I wondered how I could impact the fitness industry for Christ. I mean, I loved Jesus, I was fit. Why not? Put your faith to work, people! Then Louie Giglio emailed me: "Jimmy, in an industry where size is king, embracing your smallness is the key." At the time, he might as well have been speaking Yiddish. It took a touch of suffering to break my back and my spirit, but I get it now.

> God is under no obligation to allow our health to improve based on our effort. But somehow in our pride, we've mistaken a gift for a debt.

Dwayne, cover your ears, brother. But it really is just a barbell. Put it in the furnace. Not the furnace of hard work. That's candy. That's easy. Put it in the furnace of uncontrollable pain and disability. Trust me. You'll never know who you really are until you break. Besides, God doesn't owe us based on our effort. Blood, sweat and tears are not payment by which we can demand a return. Our bodies are broken. Workouts are a begging. Every rep a "please." Again, God is under no obligation to allow our health to improve based on our effort. But somehow in our pride, we've mistaken a gift for a debt.

In his book, *Walking with God through Pain and Suffering,* Tim Keller says that, "Suffering drives us toward God to pray as we never would otherwise. At first this experience of prayer is usually dry and painful. But if we are not daunted, and we cling to him, we will often find greater depths of experience than we thought possible."

I often stand above my bathtub—my Gethsemane—and look down. That tub, and the years, and the loss of function, and the loss of ability are the reasons I stoop as I enter your lives with this book. Today the tub is quiet, it's kept and clean, but it's where I resigned. It will always be the "dust where I worshipped."

Travail leaves a mark.
Suffering sucks.
God's sovereignty is our only solace.
And when nobody understands, you hit your knees, face to the dirt and you sing.

As I type this sentence, I've turned on my music to an old album called, *The Story*. Filled with amazing songs that walk us through the entire Bible, *The Story* has a song about the Old Testament's suffering Job; perfect note to end on...

If one more person takes my hand and tries to say they understand;
tells me there's a bigger plan that I'm not meant to see.
If one more person dares suggest that I held something unconfessed
and tries to make the dots connect from righteousness to easy street.
Who else will see my suffering as one more opportunity to educate
and help me see all my flawed theology?
If one more well-intentioned friend tries to tie-up my loose ends;
hoping to—with rug and broom—sweep awkward moments from the room...
But who am I to make demands of the God of Abraham?

And God, who are You that You would choose to answer me with mercy new?
How many more will wander passed to find me here among the ash.
Will you hold me? Will You stay so I can raise this broken praise to You?
But You were the one who filled my cup.
And You were the one who let it spill.
So blessed be Your Holy Name if you never fill it up again.
If this is where my story ends, just give me one more breath to say,
"Hallelujah."

~The Wheelhouse~

It was good for me to be afflicted so that I might learn your decrees.
— Psalm 119:71

A diving accident in 1967 left 17-year-old Joni Eareckson Tada a quadriplegic. An attractive, athletic believer, Joni had her sights set on taking life by the tail. In an interview with Crossway Books about her project *Hymns of Suffering,* Joni said, "Before my diving accident, I prayed for Jesus to do something in my life that would draw me close to Him. Then I broke my neck. And I remember thinking, 'How could you take my prayer so seriously? I didn't mean *this.*' I thought, 'God could never be trusted with another prayer again.' And yet, where else could I turn?"

Today she sees her disability as divine, and her suffering as safety. Though she grew up active, her greatest blessing in life hasn't been wellness or strength or ability, but rather has been found in sickness, sorrow, and loss. Why? Because of the arms to which they made her turn. "Suffering is meant to press us up against Jesus," she says. "My paralysis is about knowing Him better."

Joni & Friends was launched in 1979 to share the hope of the Gospel and give practical help to people impacted by disability worldwide. She and her friends have been changing communities around the globe for more than 40 years. They recently supplied their 400,000th wheelchair and Bible to those in need. One of my life's highest honors was serving Joni, alongside her team at Joni & Friends, over the span of a couple of years. One day I knelt in her office, held her hand, and she prayed for PrayFit and for things like this book to reach those impacted by disabilities. In fact, half of the proceeds from this book will go to support Joni's team in Texas and Brazil.

Her ministry is a result of the sweet, lifelong exchange between sovereign Savior and suffering saint. Dedicated to spreading the Gospel and serving those impacted by disability all around the world, those that work alongside her extend the long line of friends that connect the decades—divinely and affectionally sanctioned to join her as she continues to form her response in the most sacred of conversations.

Whether it's through her retreats for families impacted by special needs, or her curriculum for churches in need of content, Joni has made a habit out of helping people find diamonds in their disability and God's sovereignty in suffering.

Truth be told and forever bonded, the recipients of the gift of mobility may never meet Joni herself. They may never hear her high-pitched, joy-filled voice. They likely will never see her face-to-face, share a meal, or join her in song. But on their respective dusty roads of obscurity, amid languages as diverse as the cultures they represent, they look down and push the wheels of their chairs and, somehow, they touch her, and she feels it.

Joni says, "Deep trials bring the deep grace of God. Because there are more important things in life than standing up and walking. Suffering may be God's choicest tool in shaping the character of Christ in us."

Only someone who has taken her journey can say that and mean it. Imagine. To be *favored* with illness. But I realize that sounds lofty, almost impossible. At least for me it does. But to be grateful for her quadriplegia, Joni needed time.

Her eyes had not yet adjusted to the bleak nothingness, void of light. *My permanent paralysis had plummeted me into a deep, dark depression, and I was sinking quickly into despair. During the night when hospital visiting hours were over, I would violently wrench my neck back and forth on my pillow, hoping to snap it at a higher level, and so end my misery,* she writes in her book, *Beyond Suffering.*
She doesn't sound favored by her illness, does she?

But, I mean, would you be thankful and grateful and be praising God in the darkness if you had just broken your neck, and in the pitch blackness faced the reality that you would never move anything below your shoulders? Shoot. I've pitched bigger fits when the front desk agent of my local gym accidentally slept through their alarm clock.

But Joni will tell you that someone met her in the darkness. A young 17-year-old friend named Steve opened his Bible at her bedside. Reading

Ephesians 5:18-20 to her, *Instead, be filled with the Holy Spirit, singing psalms and hymns and spiritual songs...and give thanks for everything to God the Father in the name of our Lord Jesus Christ.*

"But I don't feel thankful."

"Trusting God has nothing to do with trustful feelings."

"But a life of total paralysis? It's too much."

Their exchange went on for some time.

She would later write, *I thought I was being hypocritical to thank God when I didn't feel thankful, and it would have been hypocritical to thank God only to impress others, but I was tired of being depressed. I was weary of all the self-pity, and I knew I had to start somewhere in order to move forward into life.*

The moment reminds me of a moving sermon, "Songs in the Night," where Dr. Charles Spurgeon revealed the struggle of the Christian trying to praise God in the dark: "It is easy to sing when we can read the notes by daylight, but he or she is the skillful singer who can sing when there is not a ray of light by which to read—who sings from the heart, and not from a book they can see, because they have no means of reading, save from that inward book of their own living spirit, whence notes of gratitude pour forth in songs of praise."

It's said that when a jeweler shows his best diamonds, he sets them against a black velvet backdrop; the contrast of the jewels against the dark velvet brings out the luster. In the same way, God does his most stunning work where things seem hopeless. Wherever there is pain, suffering, and desperation, Jesus is.

Joni says, "Suffering will teach you who you are. It's a textbook that will show you the stuff of which you are made. And sometimes it's not very pretty. Suffering will squeeze that out of you."
Joni hated being paralyzed, but she also hated the "suffocation of self-pity." She realized she could not continue living in such hopelessness, so

she broke. She surrendered. And millions of people across generations have been and will be blessed by the power of the Gospel because of it.

Today, after more than half a century living as a quadriplegic, it's her daily struggle with chronic pain that makes her life hard. So hard in fact that, "Chronic pain makes my quadriplegia feel like a walk in the park. I can do quadriplegia, but it's hard to do pain. I have to constantly tell my heart to go find Jesus. I talk to my pain. 'Pain, you are not going to crush me.' So I sing to Jesus. And I wish I could describe the sweetness and the intimacy that I find with my Savior. So God, bless the pain. What a harsh, severe mercy. But what a sweet one. Because it has helped me love him."

May her story be a source of perspective; a reservoir of comfort; a reminder that faith doesn't mean fitness. (Joni's story makes "faith and fitness" sound so corny and meaningless, right? I know.) But may the curtain we pull back through her example be the black velvet where God's love glitters. I think you'll find that the black velvet doesn't lead to a door. It *is* the door, one that leads to an unprecedented journey.

Books To Read by Joni:
Hymns of Suffering
Beyond Suffering

> *May her story be a source of perspective; a reservoir of comfort; a reminder that faith doesn't mean fitness.*

~ The Pool of Pain ~

"Here's what happens in times of suffering.
When the thing you've been trusting is laid to waste,
you don't suffer just the loss of that thing; you also suffer the loss
of the identity and security that it provided."
— Paul Tripp

The pool of Bethesda was known for its crowd. But not just *any* crowd. The hurting kind. The desperate kind. Max Lucado describes the scene:

"Picture a battlefield strewn with wounded bodies, and you see Bethesda. Imagine a nursing home overcrowded and understaffed, and you see the pool. Can you picture it? Jesus walking among the suffering. It was the Passover feast. People have come from miles around to meet God in the temple. Little did they know God was with the sick. Little do they know God is walking slowly, stepping carefully between the beggars, the lame, and the blind."

Why did they congregate? Well, underground springs would cause the water to bubble at the surface. It was thought that the bubbles were the visible sign of the dipping of angel wings. And if you were close enough to be the first to touch the water after the angel did, you'd be healed.

The scene sends me back to my time in Israel, Romania, and Brazil, to the lines of people waiting to visit their own Bethesda. Ladies sitting in the dirt, waving away a stubborn fly while wearing their favorite dresses; men in suits that were two sizes too big and with borrowed ties; children being carried in by grandparents that have adopted them as their own because the children's parents either ran away or passed away.

A modern-day Pool of Bethesda. They came in on their hands, wearing their Sunday best. Why? Because it was the most important day of their lives. It was the day they were to receive their first wheelchair, and likely their first Bible.

When you're suffering, you still go to the pool.

God is where you least expect Him. Fast-forward 2,000 years: if Jesus were confined to one location, where would He go? I'm not sure. Ringside at HBO boxing? Courtside seats at Madison Square Garden? The owner's box at Yankee Stadium? Maybe he'd attend the CrossFit Games, but up in the rafters to accept the point of praise from the champion.

My sinful heart doubts it. No, I double down on the belief that He'd be in hospital rooms watching kids point to where it hurts. I think He'd still be in our Bethesda.

R.C. Sproul once wrote, *For a person to be called upon to suffer is not surprising once we understand who God is*. That's powerful stuff. But "God majors in suffering," says Sproul. Jesus himself was known as the man of sorrows and the suffering servant. It's no wonder Peter said not to feel it strange if we suffer.

If God is who he says he is, there is no such thing as meaningless suffering. Whether you're reading this book as someone with chronic pain, or simply someone who wants to have a clear picture of the topic, may that set us up to accept that God is with us in our suffering, he is involved in our suffering, and sometimes he calls us to it. For some, it's a vocation.

Paul Tripp was correct. You don't just suffer the pain, but also the loss of any identity because of it. But we can find comfort in knowing that, through the travail, God is rearranging our hearts and minds to find our identity in Him, and not in whatever it is that has been taken from us or added to us through illness or loss. Whether you're there to help others or you're there because you're desperate, it's okay.

Jesus knows to find us at the pool.

~The Dark Psalm~

When you suffer and lose, that does not mean you are being disobedient to God. In fact, it might mean you're right in the centre of His will. The path of obedience is often marked by times of suffering and loss."
— Chuck Swindoll

S**uffering is sacred. It's holy ground**. It's in the grip of His robe. It's in the hole in the roof. It's in the muddy water. It's in the baggy clothes of a former leper, in the corners of Peter's regret, David's shame, and Paul's remorse. And you can be sure of one thing: it's in your pain and mine. It's also in the darkest of Psalms.

"Most Psalms of lament eventually turn," says Pastor Ajay Thomas. He's right. They eventually pivot. Change directions. And although they begin in descent and despair, they eventually ascend. At some point God shows up. But not in this Psalm. Psalm 88 begins in darkness and gets even darker.

Described as the Psalm that has no hope, experts have described Psalm 88 as, "A cellar with no stairs. A prison with no key. Absolute hell on earth. Total loneliness. Utter torment. Complete darkness."

Suffering.

In verse 11, the Psalmist begins asking questions. "Can those in the grave declare your unfailing love?" (Verse 12), "Can anyone in the land of forgetfulness talk about your righteousness?" In other words, the psalmist is asking if anything good can come out of his pain. He's crying out like a blind man in a black room with no way out and nobody to help him.

Pretty grim, right? But what a comfort to you and to me that one of the authors in the Bible held on to God so tightly that in the worst of circumstances—the kind of rock-bottom event that would eventually make its way into Holy scripture—he could cry out to God, complain to God, question God, and eventually collapse on Him.

Our dark days can remind us of the darkness that only Jesus could pierce. In fact, while the Psalmist began and ended in darkness, he wasn't *actually* alone. Only Jesus Himself experienced the kind of loneliness the Psalmist described when God turned His back on Him at Calvary. Only Jesus could call the darkness His only friend. He did that so that our sins could be forgiven and that we would never be forsaken.

Jesus became the light of the world and would eventually hang on the Cross in complete darkness, and unlike the psalmist, Jesus was completely alone. *Jesus suffered.* And in doing so, He answered the questions in verses 11 and 12 of Psalm 88:

"Can those in the grave declare your unfailing love?" (*Yes.*)
"Can they proclaim your faithfulness in the place of destruction?" (*Yes.*)
"Can the darkness speak of your wonderful deeds?" (*Yes.*)
"Can anyone in the land of forgetfulness talk about your righteousness?" (*Yes.*)

Prayers like Psalm 88 indicate God's understanding. Tim Keller says, "God knows how people speak when they're desperate; he identifies with us in our suffering."

You know, I've spent the past few years focused on helping kids impacted by special needs, and that focus is only becoming more intense. I've traveled the globe—from Israel to Bucharest to Brazil—and I've seen some hurting people. Blind, deaf, lame. No arms. No legs. No family. No water. Real hurts. Real need. Read bad. But the truth is, I've never felt closer to God than when I'm with those who are truly in need of the Gospel, in complete despair and desperate for physical and mental healing.

It's intense to imagine that the psalmist thought darkness was his only friend, but we know that God was closer. There's a reason why we sense God in the rough places and the tight spots and the lonely corners. He's where broken people go.

REFLECTION

I've always been a hard charger. I hate to lose more than I like to win. I'm emotional, sentimental, and motivated. I'm a natural worrier, I'm creative, passionate, and introverted. I'm in my head a lot. And I have a temper.

I grew up as the skinny kid in every sport. But things changed in college. In the late eighties, there was one, and only one, fitness center on the campus of Baylor University: Russell Gymnasium. The gym itself was actually a corner hole in the wall within a bigger auditorium of basketball courts, with a two-tone puke-green concrete wall that separated the outdated Universal equipment and rusty dumbbells from the courts next door. It was pretty terrible. It was awesome.

I was eighteen, the newest member of a very small band of brothers. We weren't an official group on campus by any means, these "Russell Rats." We had no membership roster, no board of directors or rules and regulations to speak of, but we were very exclusive. And although we weren't organized, we did pay our dues; "dues" of a different kind were collected daily. As far as acceptance into the group, well, it just happened. Call it a nonverbal recognition of pure heart. If you had it, you were in. And rather than Greek letters across our chest, we had chalk and sweat across our backs. There was no mistaking our crew.

And that's when my health and fitness journey began. I was serious. I remember being so happy in the gym. I'd lie back on the bench and say this motivational speech in my head: *I'm saved, forgiven, my family loves me, I'm growing, and I have an amazing future.* Then I'd hit the set and kill it until it crushed me. I did that for years. It meant so much to me that I eventually earned a master's degree in exercise physiology, landed a great gig as a writer and director at Muscle & Fitness magazine, and carried a handful of fitness books and projects on my resume. In my line of work, I was the man. I was at the top of the fitness industry.

That's what I brought to my season of suffering. But it's not all I brought.

In his book, *Suffering: Gospel Hope When Nothing Makes Sense*, Paul Tripp says, *You and I never come to our suffering empty-handed. We always drag a bag full of experiences, perspectives, desires, intentions, and decisions into our suffering. Two things I didn't know I was carrying into my physical travail that shaped how I walked through my experience: pride and unrealistic expectations.*

Pastor Tripp and I share some similar qualities. I brought not only pride and expectations to my suffering but I carried a lukewarm relationship with God into it as well. I had unconfessed sin in my heart before God and my wife, doubts in my mind and broken dreams. Suffering physically is bad. Suffering physically in the fitness industry is worse. But suffering without a good grasp of the Gospel is like sinking in quicksand while in a straitjacket. And the distance between how you feel in suffering and the ability for someone else to grasp it or understand it only adds to the misery. You can't describe it well enough for someone else to feel, and that in and of itself is torture.

Here's the deal. In true suffering, you can't fight your way out on your schedule. You can't defend yourself, help yourself, or solve it with a "10-day reset." In the mud, you quickly learn what you have based your life upon or put your trust and worth into. It exposes your misguided dependencies. It reveals a cavity, a junk drawer of empty resources you thought would get you through, because getting through has always been your thing. You just dig deep, even in the most difficult of normal circumstances, right? But these are not normal circumstances. Normal circumstances of chasing dreams, setting goals, counting calories, losing, winning, and competing with yourself are like picking flowers compared to life's real travail.

If it seems like I'm typing with a bit of a snarl, you're right. It's okay to be upset. It's alright to be angry at pain, sickness, and death. Suffering for a believer may be an instrument that God uses for his glory and our good, but don't let anyone tell you it's something you long for or hope for in your life.

Tim Keller says, *Suffering can lead to personal growth and training and transformation, but we must never see it as primarily a way to improve ourselves, because that can lead to a form of masochism; an enjoyment of ache, because we only feel virtuous when we are in pain. Instead, we must look at suffering—whatever the proximate causes—as a primary way to know God better, as an opening for serving, resembling, and drawing near to Him as never before.*

Again, what you bring to suffering is what you'll have during its seeming reign and rule as well as what you'll have either after you heal or if it never goes away. That's super critical to remember. You may come out more compassionate or more contemptuous. You could rise from the ash renewed for the most meaningful things in life or more skeptical and even sarcastic to scoff at life itself. You may be more understanding of others or it may make you resentful of those that don't seem to have a thing going "wrong" with themselves.

It will all depend on whether or not you let it break you and to which side you fall.

Tim Challies, author of Seasons of Sorrow, who recently suffered personally tragedy in the loss of his son writes, "Christians have a complex relationship to suffering. We do not wish to experience suffering.

It is not our desire, preference, or longing to go through times of pain and persecution, times of sorrow and loss. Yet we also know that God uses such experiences to accomplish significant and meaningful things within us. We know there are certain graces that bloom best in the valleys, certain fruits that ripen best in the winter, certain virtues that come to fruition most often in the shadows."

Suffering makes us see ourselves differently. We're not that big, strong, or able. You and I are far more fragile than we care to admit. Suffering humbles us, lowers our view of self, and adjusts a proper perspective of ourselves. Tim Keller says, "Suffering removes the blinders. It doesn't so much make us helpless and out of control as it shows us we have always been vulnerable and dependent on God."

My faith has never moved a mountain. Says a lot about my faith. And even says a lot about the mountain. Some people in the faith and fitness industry will tell you that obstacles are put in your path so that you can show the world it can be moved. But in reality, the real obstacles in life, the kind of true travail and suffering, are there perhaps to show the world they can't be moved; that you are small and that God allows for the limits. It's in those moments that the world hears us say, "I can't. God can. But if he doesn't, I still believe."

To celebrate God, train. To trust God, fail. To touch God, suffer.

Q: Are you a fitness enthusiast? A trainer? Runner? In what ways has suffering entered your world?

Q: Has it broken you to the point that you realize your smallness? Or are you still fighting in a way that says, "This mountain will prove to the world that it *can* be moved" when in reality, it can't unless God intervenes.

Q: How can suffering be a gift of grace?

Q: What is more powerful? Your strength or your weakness? Which one will never fail you?

Q: From your own experience, when Paul says that God's strength is made perfect in weakness, have you personally encountered areas in your life where that is becoming ever more true and clear?

> *To celebrate God, train. To trust God, fail. To touch God, suffer.*

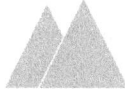

SECTION TWO
Suffering Shapes Us

Look up the word *wayward* in a thesaurus and synonyms like *stubborn, headstrong, disobedient, impossible, willful,* and *wild* make the list. Any wayward sons or daughters reading this book? Well, a wayward son is writing it. I tell you, few lyrics of any song paint as good a picture of grace in suffering as "Carry On Wayward Son" by Kansas.

Maybe you can relate. Perhaps notes of suffering, personal failure, failed health, or heartbreak, bad breaks, and mistakes make for the lyrics of your most current verse. Hopefully something you read in this section will shape your sweet spirit and help your strong soul to carry on.

"Carry on, my wayward son...
There'll be peace when you are done...
Lay your weary head to rest...
Don't you cry no more."

~Strong in the Dark~

In my own life, I think I can honestly say that out of the deepest pain has come the strongest conviction of the presence of God and the love of God."
— Elisabeth Elliot

After meeting in college, Jay and Katherine Wolf married and moved to Los Angeles to pursue careers in law and entertainment. At that time, they were living on-campus of Pepperdine University, where they were the young parents of little James.

Just three weeks before Jay was set to graduate, Katherine suffered a rupture in her brain as the result of a mass known as an arteriovenous malformation (AVM). Many of you know Jay and Katherine through their ministry and books and their powerful voices. I think in this day and age, amid the cultural, political, and health crises, theirs could be some of the most needed voices for the believing world to hear.

I was watching a video of theirs at Passion Church a few months ago, and Katherine was asked at the end of the service to pray for the viewers. She said, "I'd be happy to pray, but let me just say…."

Katherine had promising careers in entertainment, modeling, and maybe even acting. She was living in Malibu, married to a soon-to-be lawyer, and was the mother of a newborn who was filling the house with joy and life. If you've ever been to Malibu, and specifically to Pepperdine, the sunrise and sunsets dancing off the Pacific Ocean have Eden-like features and characters. Every morning seagulls sing, whales wale, and deer graze the steep, vast, manicured lawn of the campus as the mist begins to lift from the shoreline across Highway 1.

I picture Katherine squinting and grinning as she opens up her blinds to let the light in. Life was good. But as written in her book, *Hope Heals*, Katherine was rushed to UCLA Medical Center following her stroke, and one of the world's best neurosurgeons, Dr. Nestor Gonzalez, "just happened" to be on call. It was the largest AVM he had ever seen, and in the worst location. She was not expected to live, but despite the grim prognosis and the lawyer husband, he decided to take the case.

Today, half of her body is paralyzed, among other physical battles, as she and Jay continue to speak truth about suffering well—if not strong—to millions around the world.

So, when Louie Giglio asked her to pray at Passion, she said, "I'd be happy to pray, but let me just say, God gives hidden treasure in the secret places so that we may know him and live differently because of the treasure we get to take hold of and cherish and champion for the rest of our lives. That treasure—and this is a deep comfort—is only available when we are in the deep darkness. We get to hold it and let it inform how we live moving forward. That is special stuff. Don't miss it in the darkness. Get that treasure and let it change you."

God could have used Katherine Wolf to impact millions through movie roles and modeling gigs, but God chose her for the vocation of suffering. He sent her to the dark places beneath the layers of health and wealth, to the deepest recesses of pain and desperation and hollowness and pitch blackness. It was there Katherine realized that the treasure has nothing to do with the physical; be it in the world or of the body, the treasure is the promise of Jesus and His sacrifice and the knowledge that we will be with Him for all eternity.

If it needs to be repeated: you may not come out of times of suffering healed or better or having made any progress, but you do come out different. In some cases, both weaker *and* stronger. But that doesn't happen unless—as Katherine implores—we get the treasure and hold it and cherish it and champion it so that it informs and shapes how we live. It's no wonder she encourages us to suffer strong.

I tell ya, it takes real inner work to live sick. If you or someone you love is in the grip of it, this is me nodding as I type. Some people walk around with invisible chronic pain, but you'd never know it. They just glide through life with an uncommon poise. But make no mistake, the travails they endure would buckle your knees and cause most of us to fold like a chair.

The good news is that pain and suffering brought out the worst in me. That's what it does. By grace, it revealed significant cracks in my character, crevices that exposed my temper, my lust of the flesh, my little faith and little idols—not to mention my pride and self-pity. It shattered my categories. But it doesn't always work out that well. It happens only if you heed Katherine's advice and get the treasure and let it change you.

~He's No Machine~

We are healed of a suffering only by experiencing it to the full.
— Marcel Proust

If you've suffered, you're well aware that suffering isn't bound to its epicenter. The ripple effect and its incremental outward expansion goes beyond the physical origin and reaches well outside the target. Amid the tough stuff of life, you've likely been sad or worried, you've questioned God, or you've longed for a do-over. And you've probably wondered whether or not it will "always be like this" and if there's hope for a normal future. If you haven't, I, despite my delusions of strength, have.

So has Kevin Scahill.

Kevin is no machine. More than two decades ago, he was driving with his daughter along the streets of Dallas—the same streets he patrolled as a seasoned police officer—when his car was hit by a semi-truck. His daughter walked away with a few stitches; Kevin suffered a traumatic brain injury.

His speech is muddled, his breathing is labored, and his posture is as straight as a question mark. Wrapped in a makeshift brace that begins around his ankle and attaches to his belt loop, his right leg wants to go one way while his left leg is determined to go another. You and I will take 10 steps before he takes two.

I met Kevin at the Texas Joni & Friends Family Retreat, where families impacted by special needs travel for hours—and even days in some cases—to hang with friends, worship together, relax, go fishing, play games, learn about Jesus, and just have a blast. Kevin, however, isn't a camper. He's a volunteer leader. He's a servant; a humble, sweet, God-fearing, Gospel-dropping, suffering saint. The spiritual warfare he's involved in is so palpable that the friendly fire inside his heart strays to reach my pride and defeats it on impact. The longer I live and the more mistakes I make, the more I realize it's impossible to be proud in the presence of the humble.

As we stood together and welcomed families to the camp, the only thing higher than the Texas heat was the energy coming from the crew of volunteers. As they line-danced to "Footloose" in exuberant anticipation of their guests, Kevin turned to me and, with beads of sweat dripping from his brow, he said through the noise, "Jimmy, I don't want to elevate her, and I don't want to lower Christ, but Joni Eareckson Tada is the closest thing to Jesus I have ever known."

Gulp. (Pull it together, Peña.)

Each morning before the 7 a.m. prayer, Kevin could be found swimming his laps and doing his therapy. In fact, over the course of the past 20 years, he's learned how to breathe, eat, stand, talk, and walk—all for the second time. And yes, he's learned how to fight. By God's grace, he stands toe-to-toe with suffering and doesn't flinch.

I used to think that the battle raged within reps and between sets, through pumps and progress and through the welcomed blood, sweat, and tears of grit. Not so. That kind of battle is a masquerade party under the guise of pain and punishment, so write this down: If you look forward to it, it's not suffering.

I've said it before, but angels don't rejoice when we reach our fitness goals. They rejoice when a lost person chooses Christ. Truth is, the Apostle Paul disciplined his body like an athlete—not to turn heads but to change hearts. It's warfare. And from experience, *real* suffering attacks the heart and goes for the soul.

> *If you look forward to it, it's not suffering.*

I've met a warrior in Kevin who isn't going to let that happen.

When I got sick a few years ago, my grasp of my mortality tightened and my sensitivity to the brittleness of my body heightened. I came face-to-face with a certain truth: that my physical limit wasn't my personal best, like my bench press (405 pounds) or my squat (550 pounds)—imposters disguised as my potential. I list them only to help illustrate that those mountain-top moments didn't represent my personal best. No, the most strenuous minute I've ever filled came when I realized I would never attempt to best them.

Bodily stewardship is truly an ever-growing *tension* for me, as if each ticking second of the clock represents the loosening stitch of the fabric of my physical self. I mean, I know I'm withering. I know I'm wasting away, and yet I am called to fight. I'm called to steward. I'm called here on Earth to nurse my dying shell with a heavenly mind.

Guys, I'm fighting. Clawing and reaching. I may not be as able as ever, but I still *rage against the dying of the light.* Knowing Heaven is in view and by faith it will make sense of Earth, I'm trying to fill the minutes and days with the kind of physical stewardship that allows me to do what God asks.

The fact of the matter is, I've lost health, friends, dignity. Personally and physically, I've lost my grip on a lot. I have irreversible bone loss and disk degeneration, and unrecoverable colon function. I have trouble sleeping. Working on getting my mind right. On the shallow end, my muscle will never thrive like it once did. I can't run, twist, or jump. But my physical state doesn't determine my call to steward the body God gave me. So I keep trying. Fighting.

Spiritually, well, that's far more important. I need clear eyes and a clean heart. New morning mercy. I'm growing in grace because of how much I need it. My sin is met by amazing grace. He's holding on to me. It says in Psalm 139:14, *I will praise you for I am fearfully and wonderfully made.* Let's look at the verse for a second.

> *I'm called here on Earth to nurse my dying shell with a heavenly mind.*

"I will praise you." In other words, the outflow, the attention, the adoration, and the praise is appropriately *leaving* the Psalmist. Nowhere in that verse is there any sense of a longing for attention from the writer.

"Fearfully and wonderfully." Adverbs that divinely and miraculously qualify the verb *made.*

Made. Created, done, finished, completed, approved. We don't add or subtract to the process.

Fearfully and wonderfully made. In other words, completely dependent upon—nothing until made into something. The created (that's us) releasing all honor and glory to the Creator (God) for the most basic of reasons: being nothing without Him. Training doesn't improve it; sickness doesn't diminish it. The fact that we're fearfully and wonderfully made says something profound about us, but not nearly as profound as what it says about God.

Our workouts are a *begging.* Our workouts are an *ovation.* You and I aren't "creating" when we train. We're not making or building, and we're most certainly not improving God's work. But every move, every step, every rep, set, and stretch is a glorious unfolding and an instantaneous, miraculous unveiling. Just...not of us. A.W. Tozer says, "The worshipping heart does not create its Object."

Frankly, nobody reading this sentence—or anyone who ever lived, for that matter—has ever physically traveled beyond their God-given limits. Nobody. Even our best workout is an awesome display of weakness. Reaching God-given limits is a humbling orientation. Each day, if I need to remind myself of just how big God is and how weak and small I am, I just do my best. We are not made of steel, but dust. Make perfect in weakness. We don't know strong yet.

And while that might seem like a slap in the face to the motivational speaker who claims we can push beyond limits, the truth is, we never exceed our limits. We merely—if rarely—find them. And I like to think that in finding our limits, we meet God.

> *Even our best workout is an awesome display of weakness. Reaching God-given limits is a humbling orientation. Each day, if I need to remind myself of just how big God is and how weak and small I am, I just do my best.*

"Mortals, born of woman,
are of few days and full of trouble.
They spring up like flowers and wither away;
like fleeting shadows, they do not endure.
Do you fix your eye on them?
Will you bring them before you for judgment?
Who can bring what is pure from the impure? No one!
A person's days are determined;
you have decreed the number of his months
and have set limits he cannot exceed.
(Job 14: 1-5)

~Love Me Tender~

There are none so tender as those who have been skinned themselves.
— C.H. Spurgeon

The genius use of the word *tender* in the quote above isn't lost on me—showing compassion because you're sensitive to the pain.

It's well documented that in his bedroom, Charles Spurgeon had a plaque on the wall with Isaiah 48:10 that read: *I have chosen thee in the furnace of affliction.* He once wrote, *Men will never become great in divinity until they become great in suffering. There are none so tender as those who have been skinned themselves. Those who have been in the chamber of affliction know how to comfort those who are there. Do not believe that any man will become a physician unless he walks the hospital; and no one will become a comforter unless he lies in it and has to suffer himself.* (Christian George, The Spurgeon Center.)

He would know. Spurgeon suffered from myriad mental and physical hardships: kidney inflammation, gout, and depression, just to name a few of his struggles.

Cancer survivor and medical director of the Bellevue Hospital Center, Dr. Eric D. Manheimer, said in the *New York Times*, "No amount of doctoring can prepare you for being a patient. If anything, it's that recognition of vulnerability as well as expertise that makes me a better doctor today." Something tells me Dr. Manheimer would agree with Spurgeon. After all, it was Spurgeon's illness—not his fitness—that assured him of God's grip on him and God's love for him. "You must go through the fire if you would have sympathy with others who tread the glowing coals," Spurgeon says.

"I, the preacher of this hour, beg to bear my witness that the worst days I have ever had have turned out to be my best. When God has seemed most cruel to me, he has been most kind. If there is anything in this world for which I would bless him more than for anything else, it is for pain and affliction. I am sure that in these things the richest, tenderest love has been manifested to me. Love letters from heaven are often sent in black-edged envelopes."

Wow. Right? The dirt where his face sank was an altar. He worshipped where he wept. He saw it as guided, directed affection. First *to* him and then *from* him. His tender pain was a love note that he would read and send back. For the Christian in the fitness industry reading this, suffering is a love letter. First to you, then from you. A mystery novel, then a psalm.

Now, I don't mean to put words into his mouth, but this old Elvis song comes to mind. As a modern-day psalm to his God, I think for Spurgeon it would be just about perfect...

Love me tender,
love me long,
take me to Your heart.
For it's there that I belong,
and we'll never part.

> *For the Christian in the fitness industry reading this, suffering is a love letter. First to you, then from you. A mystery novel, then a psalm.*

~The Weak Applause~

"When you become consumed by God's call on your life, everything will take on new meaning and significance. You will begin to see every facet of your life—including your pain—as a means through which God can work to bring others to Himself."
— Charles Stanley

If you've read my books or have seen "The PrayFit Story," you know by now that Louie Giglio once put me in my place. I was working for the leader in fitness publishing when I asked Louie how I could make an impact on the fitness industry for Christ. He replied, "Embrace your smallness."

You'll have to watch the video for how that turned out, but in his book, *I Am Not but I Know I AM,* Louie writes, *You and I are tiny. Among us, the strongest of the strong can be felled in one faltering heartbeat. We are fleeting mortals. Frail flesh. Little specks. If this fact makes you just a tad bit uncomfortable, you're not alone. Invariably, when I talk about the vastness of God and the cosmos, someone will say, 'You're making me feel bad about myself and making me feel really, really small' (as if that's the worst thing that could happen). But the point is not to make you feel small, rather to help you see and embrace the reality that you are small... Really, really small.*

When you're aware of your smallness, when you become aware of your dependence and your neediness, you actually come to life. There is something liberating about waking up each day knowing you're not nearly as strong as you think you are.

I tell ya, the more I've seen suffering in the world, among friends and in my own life, the more I'm convinced that God wants my heart renewed by His grace and for me to obey His commands and love others. Simple as that. Like those much wiser than me, I believe we were made to worship. But I have fooled many people over the course of my life into supposing that when I train physically,

> *There is something liberating about waking up each day knowing you're not nearly as strong as you think you are.*

"I'm worshipping." I've even written poems about it and published chart-topping books with that theme.

And while I do know there have been times when that's been true, when my heart and mind have been in His presence as I perform a certain stretch or when I'm on the bike in tune to His will, I also know I'm full of nonsense in so many ways. And nobody knows it more than the God of the universe that I mock when I secretly, privately, and oftentimes publicly glory in my own physical accomplishments.

Truth is, God doesn't need my lift or my grit. He doesn't need my squat, my flexibility, my PR, my competitive heart. He doesn't need me. He doesn't need me strong, fast, thick, or thin. He doesn't need me lighter, quicker, more intense or less. He doesn't even need me around. He doesn't even need me healthy or healed. And I know I don't deserve any of it. As William Munny, played by Clint Eastwood in *Unforgiven*, said so beautifully, "Deserve's got nothin' to do with it." That's right, William Munny. You don't earn your body. It's a gift.

And somehow in His immeasurable grace and mercy, He just wants me and loves me. He wants a relationship with me. He died on the cross and made the sacrifice for all my sins, so I don't have to work my way to Heaven, but I simply need to accept Him by grace through faith.

The most generous thing we can do with our suffering and/or good health is offer it up as a living sacrifice because of the sacrifice He became for us. And our living sacrifice has *nothing* to do with our performance in some gym, how well we plan our meals, or in the byproducts of our diligence. But our living sacrifice has *everything* to do with hearts being changed by the grace of God and in the spiritual change that occurs with and through our bodies as a result. God will glorify our bodies. That's not our job.

Our job is to follow Jesus, encourage others to do the same, and "for the glory of God" we look after ourselves in the process. God cares more about our bodies than we do. Imagine that. He made them, He knows we need them, and someday He'll heal them.

And I know I've said it before, but we're very stoppable. We have God-given abilities with God-given limits. And that's a God-given compliment. What do we do with a compliment God gives us? We accept it. And our response, in the form of our highest effort, is one of the ways we simply say thank you for the gift of limitation. But we can never hook our hope to health. We should never base our joy on a weight we can lift.

In his book, *The Road to Character*, David Brooks describes our current culture in a way that few dare. *As I look around, the same messages are everywhere. You are special. Trust yourself. Be true to yourself. Commencement speeches are larded with the same clichés: Follow your passion. Don't accept limits. You are so great. This self-centeredness leads in several unfortunate directions. It leads to selfishness. It leads to pride. It leads to a capacity to ignore your imperfections and inflate your virtues; constantly seeking recognition and painfully sensitive to any snub to the status we feel we have earned for ourselves.*

As I look at the fitness industry, and even the "faith & fitness" corner of it, it seems we are hellbent on assuring one another that it's all about being abundantly comfortable in our own skin, to the point that we dramatize and sensationalize our unfiltered posts in the anticipation of the applause for our brutal honesty and the risk of being exposed as merely human.

From experience, such attempts at recognition rival the desire for the same kind of "likes" we covet for our most beloved pics, attractive angles, and best sides. We're glory hounds. Praise junkies. Self-trusted wannabes. Oh, but we want *everyone* to accept the mantra that we're unstoppable because we are "enough" and that we can do anything we set our minds to.

"I just wish other women knew how amazing they were. Straighten out that crown, girl!" Or, "I just wish other men knew how many mountains they could move if they just believed in themselves."

Hogwash. This is the false gospel of self-trust. And the travail of life will sniff that out and expose it for what it's worth, which isn't much. Trust me, we are not that awesome and that mountain ain't gonna budge, no matter how hard you push yourself. The travail of chronic illness and suffering will expose the falsehood of self like nothing else. If I can ascend into the gym or studio—the shallow periphery that I know as well as any and better than most—when was the last time you and I praised and applauded God for His allowance of our limits? Forget our basements, what about for our ceilings? Limits are both above and below. Our health has a purpose and a limit. Same goes for our sufferings. Purpose and limits.

Whether it's from a hospital bed or a squat rack, we're mixing it up with the best that life can throw at us. We do our best to put up our dukes and slip its jab, but it's a fight we will eventually lose. I know it's a blow to the body, but health is a losing battle. Thankfully, gracefully, our spiritual battle was fought and won only when He said, "It is finished." And if the world hears that as an admission of weakness, they're right. Only, we know it as applause. An applause that echoes off the bottom floor of our despair to the rooftops of our ability.

When we own our weakness, we applaud God.

***

In the Old Testament, when God says to Job, *Dress for action like a man; I will question you and you will make it known to me,* (Job 38:3) God isn't telling Job how great his manhood is. Actually, this is God telling Job how great his manhood *isn't.* God is putting Job in his place.

Pastor Paul Tripp says that God tells Job to "put his best person pants on" because He is going to ask him a couple of questions. See, God is drawing a line of distinction between a creature and a Creator. God says, *Where were you when I laid the foundations of the earth? Tell me if you have understanding. Who determined the measurements? You surely know.* (v. 4)

Job was a humble, godly man who ultimately found God to be fair and just (even in suffering). In fact, at the end of the book, we find Job having a deeper relationship with God because of his trials. It's been said that Job is a book that examines how a Christian can sustain a close relationship with the Lord in the midst of severe travail. I find it fascinating that after all Job suffered, the loss of his family and bodily function—after all of that, God showed him Himself.

Job was unaware of the discussion between God and Satan concerning him. The invisible warfare surrounding Job's suffering is a powerful lesson, and a reminder as you and I try to embrace God's purposes for the things He allows in our lives. He didn't give Job any specific reason or justification for allowing him to suffer, but simply gave Job a glimpse of Himself in the heavenly places.

Alistair Begg says that Job, in his extremely trying circumstances, cried for the Lord. The longing desire of an afflicted child of God is to see his Father's face once more. The first and foremost cry is, "Oh, that I knew where I might find *Him*, who is my God, that I might come even to His seat!" God's children run home when the storm comes. Nothing teaches us about the preciousness of the Creator as much as when we learn the emptiness of everything else.

Does your suffering or your fitness or your general health as a dependent, created being help produce awe, wonder, and worship inside you? Or does it produce a desire for you to be worshipped, for others to be in awe of your story and in wonder of your achievements? God was doing for Job what we need to happen for us. Here's the picture God was painting: *I'm God, you're not. Get dressed. Lift some weights. Get pumped. Feel the fullness of your manhood! Ready? Good. Because in all your "human" ability, you can't answer Me.*

Awe, wonder, worship. That's what all this is about; to *enable* us to look up while being face down. The fitness industry—and even the "faith & fitness" industry—wants you to think it's about you, how *you're* enough. But in truth, guys, it's when we realize that God is God and we're not that we actually get it; that our greatest achievements in life (especially our perception of physical strength) are distractions if we allow them to be, especially when we buy the lie that we deserve anything. The line of distinction between the created (us) and the Creator (God) will never be crossed.

Your blog is not the 5th gospel. Your fitness books are not divine. Your nutrition advice is not manna from above. You don't have a monopoly on suffering. Getting up off the canvas is a gift of grace, not a chance to gloat about grit. So when you wipe the dust off your back, try not to pat.

~Dark Place, High Praise~

It's the trust in God, not the explanations from God, that is the pathway through suffering.
— Ray Ortlund

D avid was no stranger to caves. From the darkest place came his highest praise. Like you perhaps, he was no stranger to pain, adversity, and suffering. I can just hear the faint echo of water as it drops around him. Every few hours he looks and listens, wondering if the coast is clear. Among other hardships, when David wrote Psalm 57, King Saul was trying to kill him (1 Sam 24). But the young shepherd did what sheep need to do and cried out loudly to the only One who could help him, the only One who could hold him, and the only One *with* him in his refuge until the storm passed.

From the darkness he wrote: *...I've run to you for dear life. I'm hiding out under your wings until the hurricane blows over. I call out to High God, the God who holds me together. (v.1-3) I'm ready, God...ready from head to toe, ready to sing, to raise a tune. (v.7,8) I'm thanking you, God, out loud...the deeper your love, the higher it goes; every cloud is a flag to your faithfulness.* (v.9,10)

Pastor Levi Lusko says, "The largest pain calls for the loudest praise." If David's cave teaches us anything, I hope it's these things:

1) You and I have permission to hurt.
2) We need to go through our trials with a spirit of enthusiasm that characterizes our suffering.
3) It's best to bring our pain to the One who can do something about it.

Everyone with me? Someone you know and love—and that someone may be in your morning's mirror—needs to read that list.

Looking back 25 years, I'd often ask Loretta to turn up the music from the other room to ready my heart for my training. But during the years of my travail, I begged her each day to turn up the music from the other room to drown out the sound caused by the pain of my infirmity. Same music, same body, different faith. Perhaps like you today, my spirit of enthusiasm characterized my suffering.

Guys, we have permission to hurt. We have Biblical examples of those that hurt so deep—physically, spiritually, emotionally—they wailed. Like me, like you, suffering (invisible or otherwise) draws it out of us. It might not be pretty, but it can be the first sound of worship.

We may not understand God's specific purposes for the suffering we face. As Alistair Begg points out, however, ignoring suffering does not work, nor does suffering in and of itself bring us closer to God. Instead, the right way to deal with suffering is to bow under the sovereignty of God's purposes and see our circumstances through the lens of the cross. Only then can we trust God's plan amid difficulty, even without seeing the whole picture. We need to take refuge in Him.

The safest place for David to go until his storm passed was a cave. Some days I want to join him. I want to duck my head as I step inside and ask the man whose heart I want to please scoot over. I then lean my back against the wall, slide down, sit, and hide. Best part is, when he starts to sing, I know the words. You do too. The end of Psalm 57 is a familiar praise. If you're in here with us—if suffering calls for the cave—this is me scooting over for you. From the darkest place comes our highest praise. In fact, I think David is about to sing. I say we join him.

We exalt Thee. We exalt Thee. We exalt Thee, O God. Be thou exalted, O God, above the heavens; let your glory be over all the earth.

Perhaps like you today, my spirit of enthusiasm characterized my suffering.

~Posture Is Everything~

To become who we want we often have to endure what we hate.
To receive what we long for we often have to release what we love.
— Tim Challies

"He was right," I said to myself. Up until that moment, we had walked all the major tourist spots and spent time listening to very knowledgeable guides. I'd seen an ancient city, dipped my feet in the Dead Sea, and stood at the Western Wall. The Holy Land was everything and more, and the Bible came to life in ways I never thought possible. But as we approached what is considered to be the tomb where Jesus was buried, I remembered something Max Lucado once wrote: *You have to stoop.*

As an old fitness expert, I can tell you that *posture is everything.* I probably can't count how many times I wrote about posture in the magazine. I assure you that some of the best advice I ever gave was that no matter the lift—with few exceptions—in order to perform at your best and put yourself in the best mechanical advantage possible, never collapse your spine. Keep your chest up, abs in tight, back flat, and head neutral.

Pastor Paul Tripp once asked, "What will you do with Easter?" He related it to issues of life, money, relationships, and troubles.

What a powerful question for us in the fitness industry. If not about Easter, what will we do with our health when the storms of life arise? What will we do when we're tempted to gloat, to boast, to pat ourselves on the back? What will we do?

What will we do when we get sick? Like, really sick. What will we do when our dreams of gains, of glorious pain, of wondrous work—when the welcome pursuit of fitness is denied us? What will we do? What will we do when the status call on social media stokes our fear of missing out?

What will we do when our loss of muscle, our gain of bodyfat, our diminishing bone mass, our elevated resting heart rate, our unrelenting atrophy, our irreversible disease progression, or our unmistakable loss of strength testify to the truth that we are made of dust, not iron.

When we peer into the empty grave, that's the lens through which everything else in life can be seen, even our bodies. And as fitness people, as hard chargers, as mile runners, as record breakers, as goal makers, and as broken-down, out-of-the-game lifters like me, the empty tomb is full of grace and joy and relief. The thought of His victory eternally exceeds our loss or gains in this vapor-quick life.

But where was I? Ah, yes. The tomb. Max assured me that you can walk up to it upright, but in order to enter, you have to stoop. And he was right. The opening to the tomb where Jesus was buried is low. You can't be proud. You can't be upright. Unlike the posture of an athlete, you can't stay neutral. Feel free to do this as you read the sentence, but you have to look down, drop your head, collapse the back, bend the knee. For us to be near Him, we have to stoop. And when we do, we find Him doing the same for us. Whether into caves, tombs, or hospital rooms, suffering will make you stoop.

REFLECTION

Kevin Skahill once wrote me a letter. An *actual* letter. The kind that took a card, an envelope and stamps. But if you know Kevin, you know it took a lot more than that. Sparing his life, the collision took his speech, his gait, his coordination and motor skills. Following his brain injury, he taught himself how to walk. (And now he's teaching me.) As angels are prone, Kevin demonstrates more thoughtfulness in a day than I show in a lifetime. On the front of the card, Hallmark said, "Just a little reminder in case you forgot." Divine irony given that Kevin's memory was shattered. But Kevin, an acronym savant, assembles more encouragement and gospel goodness than anything you or I will read on social media this day. He writes,

Jimmy,

> ***Pray Until Something Happens***
> ***Stop Worrying and Pray***
> ***Fully Rely On God.***
> ***Jesus, Others, You.***
> *I love you Jimmy.*

I'm not sure how long it took Kevin to write that much, but I can tell you this much, I'll never forget it. He also sent along a poem. You already read it at the end of section one: *When God wants to.* And while the original author remains anonymous, I read it as if I were listening to Kevin as he struggles to form each handwritten word. By all means, go back and read it again. The poem is so rich and deep and meaningful and complex that I can't put it down. But it's not for the faint of heart. In a nutshell, God can do whatever He wants. He knows what He's doing as He shapes us into those that resemble himself.

Q: How is God shaping you? Is it through pain and suffering? Is it through the eyes of someone you know and love who is going through a tough patch?

Q: You'll never see who you really are when you're fit and healthy, but when you're on the anvil of true suffering. How does that shape your perspective of your pursuit of health?

Q: If you're in the fitness industry, perhaps you're beginning to realize that while you love your sport or activity, unless it's shaping your soul, it's meaningless. Part of being shaped by God is learning to rely on Him fully. How do you know if you're being shaped through your efforts?

SECTION THREE
Suffering Sends Us

I recently returned from a mission's trip to Brazil. I accompanied the Texas branch of Joni and Friends to help distribute Bibles and wheelchairs—a life-changing trip. Pastor Melo was our Brazil-based contact; he's fluent in sign language. What's the sign for the most amazing man I've ever met? And then there was Will—brilliant. He spent his vacation from from his day job of designing upscale men's clothing to build wheelchairs from the ground up. And then there was Marcelo. Nearly blind and practically non-verbal, he was from Brazil and a classic rock madman. The list goes on. I plan to go back. At the tail end of the trip, we had the chance to visit Christ the Redeemer.

According to Wikipedia, the Christ the Redeemer statue weighs 635 metric tons and stands 98 feet high; the arms stretch 92 feet. Overlooking the city of Rio de Janeiro, Christ the Redeemer is a symbol of Christianity across the world and has become a cultural icon of both Rio de Janeiro and Brazil.

Interestingly, as we approached, I noticed what many before me have noted: The statue of Jesus had blind eyes. They were almost…cold. Mind you, we had just come from a week of watching kids receive their first wheelchairs and parents their first Bibles. We had been eyewitnesses to families being prayed for while their children were held by loving therapists and pastors. We had been looking into the face of Jesus all week. So this, as beautiful and momentous as it was, actually felt a little less like a hospital and more like an amusement park. Nothing against the one of the world's seven wonder of the world, but it just didn't feel like a miracle.

As I stood at the base of the statue, so many stories ran through my heart. Cue the masterpiece score from Rocky by Bill Conti. Seriously, all of my love, all of my hopes, all of my work and words, my sentimental foolishness, my heartaches and loss of health and renewed focus on disability—all of it rushed up with me to the top of that mountain in Brazil.

Then, looking up as I caught my breath—although the eyes were blind and the stone was cold—I enjoyed the moment very much. And why not? I knew Jesus was in the church back in Curitiba. I knew He was in the heart of Becky Ellis, the leader of the entire outreach. He was in the walk of Marcelo, the mind of Will, and in the hands of Pastor Melo. And I knew for certain that He was in the faces of the kids back in the disability department at my church. I have seen Him in Jordan, Brynn, Jennifer, Emma, Sage, and redheaded Matthew.

Joni Eareckson once wrote, "It is what we do with our bodies (not how well they function) that allows us to offer them as sacrifices. Even when our bodies do not or cannot move, they reflect the glory of God's image, acceptable in His sight." Driving down the mountain, I wasn't leaving Jesus, I was going *to* Him; to my life's work and calling. Leaning into every turn, I soaked it in. I was being sent. I was descending toward my second mountain.

~The Unprecedented Journey~

Pain insists upon being attended to. God whispers to us in our pleasures, speaks in our consciences, but shouts in our pains. It is his megaphone to rouse a deaf world.
— C.S. Lewis

Scroll through Scripture and you'll read that she did what Jacob, David, and the suffering Job couldn't do. Just run through the Bible and find as many people as possible who hurt physically—one woman did exactly what each of them would have done in an instant.

Having suffered for years with an issue that condemned her as an unwanted and unclean outcast, doctors couldn't heal her, and her family disowned her. She was out of money, out of her mind, and out of choices, so she got up out of despair. Head down, she mustered strength of heart and elbowed her way through the crowd as she uttered those most precious and powerful words of hope: *"If I can just touch the hem of His garment."*

Only the deeply hurting make that kind of journey or think those words or take that kind of risk. Max Lucado says, "A healthy woman never would have appreciated the power of touching the hem of His garment. Storms make us take unprecedented journeys."

Peter was another who did what desperate people do. Many preachers and writers have examined the story of Peter walking on water, but I think the scene is worth another look for our purposes. As you know, the storm was more than they could handle, but when Jesus came strolling across the water, Peter got out of the boat. Fearing for his life, he called out to Jesus, and Jesus said, "Come." Next thing we know, Peter did a Peter Pan into the storm and did the impossible.

Now, I'm not the first person, nor will I be the last, to point out that Peter likely would not have gotten out of the boat without the storm. Some scholars say Peter would have marveled at what he saw; nobody would dispute that Peter would have been in absolute awe. Perhaps he and the others would have stood there with jaws wide open and eyes to match. We don't know. But I agree that he would not have had the urgency to leave his circumstances. Remember, *storms make us take unprecedented journeys*. Let me say it again, Peter doesn't get out of the boat without the storm. Suffering will drive you to God like nothing else. From my experience, no amount of good health will drop you like real pain. Fitness isn't tough enough to make you do that. You need something stronger.

Ever taken one? Maybe you're like me and you're on one now. Are you hurting physically? Perhaps you've been dealing with pain unknown to most, but like the woman or Peter, something invisible and unforeseen has clouded your life or is threatening it. Or maybe you're healthy and able and you've willfully and knowingly neglected your body as a fearfully woven gift. The consequences have caught up to you and they're waiting for you at the door, along with the thugs named Fear and Regret.

Something has hit you—whether by surprise or otherwise—and you're left with a bridge to cross. Your body has broken or is breaking, and things aren't functioning properly. Your travail is unmistakable and insurmountable, and while people walk by you as they live out their lives, you summon every last drop of grace inside of you to simply stand up and take a step. You sing what Paul Tripp writes:

> *Peter doesn't get out of the boat without the storm. Suffering will drive you to God like nothing else. From my experience, no amount of good health will drop you like real pain. Fitness isn't tough enough to make you do that. You need something stronger.*

Weakness is my lot.
Suffering is my prison.
You have chained me to frailty.
I cannot break free.
But this prison is your workroom.
and I am your clay.
You are not a jailer.
You are a potter.
I have not been condemned.
I am being molded.

Whoever you are and whatever your needs, make no mistake...Jesus knows the hurt and your heart. There's no pain or scar He won't understand, so bring it all. Do like Peter and risk it. Take it. Like the woman, get up. Limp through the crowd. Crawl to safety. The Bible says that many people were pressing against Jesus when He asked, "Who touched me?" (Mark 5:30), which means that while many people actually touched Jesus on the road that day, only one *truly* reached.

~"God Will Have to Build This Chair"~

"Compassion asks us to go where it hurts, to enter into the places of pain, to share in brokenness, fear, confusion, and anguish."
— Henri J.M. Nouwen

Where the Beautiful Gate in the ancient city was exactly, I'm not sure. I've been to Israel a couple of times, and somewhere beneath two centuries of life is the entrance near Solomon's porch, where Peter and John healed the lame man.

Max Lucado describes the scene this way:

"The needy man saw the apostles, lifted his voice, and begged for money. They had none to give, yet still they stopped. Peter and John looked straight at him and said, 'Look at us!' (Acts 3:4) They locked their eyes on his with such compassion that 'he gave them his attention, expecting to receive something from them.' (v.5) Peter and John issued no embarrassed glance, irritated shrug, or cynical dismissal but an honest look."

When I began serving in the special needs department at our church, I admit I was a bit startled and a little timid. Some of the pain and suffering I witnessed caused my throat to tighten. Using just her eyes and a look, special needs pioneer Pastor Gina Spivey would urge me to, "Suck it up, Peña." She is as natural with those impacted by disabilities as I am with breathing. Over the years, she's taught me that not everyone with special needs is in pain, but from my own experience, many are. And for some, it's bad. It's not for the faint of heart. Disability is not easy on the eyes.

When I was in Romania, I would often escort therapists outside as they received their next patient. One girl in particular who was brought to the Joni and Friends outreach stands out in my mind. She was lying across the back seat of a car. Her face was puffy and pale. She was drooling and moaning. Her face was so swollen I couldn't tell if her eyes were open or closed.

A tiny tube designed to remove fluid from her lungs every hour was in her nose and taped to her face. I noticed that she was dressed for winter while the rest of us were in t-shirts. She will never walk, talk, play with friends, hold a book, or meet a boy. I struggled to hold it together. Where was Gina when I needed her?

Catching only bits and pieces of my interpreter's broken English, I came to realize the woman who brought the child was her grandmother. The young girl's parents had died a few years earlier, and the man who brought them wasn't the dad, just the driver; the taxi driver. Which explains why—as everyone else was working to carefully transfer the girl inside the facility—he was leaning against the hood to light another cigarette. Meter running, I suppose.

I'll never forget standing behind the curtain with physical therapist Colleen, as she surveyed the rows of a hundred donated wheelchairs and random parts, one hand on her hip and the other covering her mouth. I don't know how I can help this little girl. God will have to build this chair."

> *She will never walk, talk, play with friends, hold a book, or meet a boy. I struggled to hold it together.*

I was witnessing compassion. Colleen gave up her vacation and paid her own way to join a ragtag team of volunteers in the distant outreaches of Bucharest. Without her brilliant, bio-mechanical mind, the people in need would not be measured correctly for their chairs. And without her heart, the little girl from the back seat of a rented taxi would not have been truly "seen."

A modern-day Peter and John, Colleen saw this little girl for the child of God she was and went to work to make it a little easier for her caregivers to get her around. If the grandmother ever describes Jesus to her family, she could very well describe Him as a middle-aged woman in scrubs and thick glasses who spent a lot of time making sure the footrests would accommodate growing, paralyzed legs.

That was Colleen. Military units have words to describe people like Colleen: brave, trusted, equipped, selfless, and compassionate. "Compassion asks us to go where it hurts," writes Henri J.M. Nouwen, "to enter into the places of pain, to share in brokenness, fear, confusion, and anguish. Compassion challenges us to cry out with those in misery, to mourn with those who are lonely, to weep with those in tears. Compassion requires us to be weak with the weak, vulnerable with the vulnerable, and powerless with the powerless. Compassion means full immersion in the condition of being human."

I've learned that the root meaning for the word *compassion* is being somewhere "in the bowels." The belly. The gut. The bowels I understand were once thought of as the seat of "love and pity," and an ancient word that describes the impact to someone's *deepest* parts. I have a sense it's where we get the phrase, "a gut feeling." And that day, my gut told me that a little girl who couldn't walk, speak, or see was going to receive a newly constructed wheelchair—no matter what.

You Can Spot a Fake

Back in my old fitness magazine days, we would often use fake weights on photo shoots to help save the models from wear and tear. The weight would need to resemble the workout plan's prescription, of course, but in order to get all of the shots over the course of a day or two, we needed the load on the bar to appear as 400 pounds but really be half that. The sweat on the brow was real, but the look on the face was an act. (I would know.) I would call for the model to "grit your teeth" and "squint the eyes" or "smile through the pain." Not only was I the resident fitness director, but I became an expert in facial expressions.

Reminds me that in the old city, the Beautiful Gate that led to Solomon's temple was likely a very popular place for the blind, the lame, as well as for con artists to congregate. Some sat there each day in desperate need of anything that someone could give. Others were there to swindle all they could get.

I tell ya. I've been to every stop along this faith and fitness road. I've seen just about everything. I've seen the healthy body stage, the stewardship phase, and the self-worth craze. I've seen congregations turned into runways where authors like me could strut. I've been around long enough to know what's real.

Anyway, a few hours later, we were again outside on the dirt road, about to lay that sweet girl into the back seat as we tried to fit her custom-made wheelchair into the trunk of the cab. Unsure of the circumstances this little patient was going back to, Colleen—exhausted both mentally and physically—was under the arm of a teammate who was praising her work.

Per tradition, we needed a photograph of the moment. We placed the sweet child and her new chair up against the wall and asked Colleen and others to surround her. When it came time for me to snap the pic, Colleen tried to smile. But she couldn't. Tears raced from the corners of her eyes to the corners of her mouth. I suppose I could have asked her to "smile through the pain," but I know a fake smile when I see one.

Lowering the camera down from my eyes, I stood there, realizing that God's antidote for people in dire need can come in many forms, even in the form of washed-up weightlifters and wannabe writers like me. Beautiful gates, it seems, can be found in every corner of the world. You just have to find them. You may have to step out of the shadow of the squat rack, social media, and the perfect filters, but when you do, you may just find yourself walking alongside Peter, John, and Colleen. And if you find someone in pain or need, you just need to follow their example. Stop, look, and help. I'm not sure how an old fitness fanatic can become a disability advocate, but I think it has something to do with grace.

We ended up getting a beautiful group picture with everyone surrounding the little girl we had the humble privilege of serving. But we also wanted one of her alone. And when everyone stepped back for me to take the shot, I like to think she smiled.

~Some People~

"And looking up to heaven, He sighed..."
— Mark 7:34

Down the street from our condo in Los Angeles sits a row of our top stops. We have our friends at Trader Joe's, our local Italian diner where John the owner greets every table with the day's specials and an update about his kids. And then we have our UPS Store. They know me well there. They'll even check my box when I forget my key. Total VIP. Around here, I'm known. *Fuhgeddaboudit.*

Last week on my usual walk, I came upon caution tape and sawdust. *UPS is temporarily around the corner. We are making some necessary upgrades.*

New mailboxes? That's probably what they're doing. The place *was* rundown. More room for the oversized copier in the lobby area? I bet that's it. As I was imagining the obvious possibilities, the manager on duty interrupted my thoughts:

"Yeah, some people said something and complained that we weren't up to standards, so here we go."

"Standards?"

"Yeah, ADA, something about disabilities. Whatever. Gotta do what ya gotta do, am I right?"

"Right," I said uncommittedly.

He disappeared into the back, and I began my walk home carrying boxes of heavy irony. While improving the aesthetics would have been fine, the store was indeed not ADA compliant. Basically, if you were a wheelchair user, you would have no way of entering the front door. The very spot I've been shipping out goods and materials for over a decade wasn't special-needs friendly. His words bounced around my brain: "Some people said something."

Arguably my favorite stories in the Bible are the ones that have anonymous heroes. From the generous widow to the Samaritan to the friends that tore through the roof, the unnamed always seem to be the ones that make a difference. As Alistair Begg says, "The work of the Gospel is undertaken, not by names and significant popular individuals, but by a vast anonymous throng. Unknown to us. Known to God."

"...There **some people** brought to him a man who was deaf and could hardly talk, and they begged Jesus to place his hand on him. After he took him aside, away from the crowd, Jesus put his fingers into the man's ears. Then he spit and touched the man's tongue. He looked up to heaven and with a deep sigh said to him, "Ephphatha!" (which means "Be opened!")." (Mark 7:32-34 *emphasis mine*)

A few things from this story in the book of Mark are, to me, both caution tape and sawdust. First, *some people* that brought the man to the one performing miracles were given no credit. Nameless. Awesome in obscurity. If this were a Broadway show, they would be the extras in case the extras got sick. These days, that probably wouldn't fly.

Take me for instance. I'd be like, *"Hey, uh, Gospel writer Mark? If you're taking notes, name's Jimmy, last name Peña. That's P, as in...uh... Paul; E, as in Everyone will know me now; N, as in Not gonna lie, this feels pretty good..."* You get the point.

We don't know if Jesus gave away kudos to his friends, but we do know that he took the man *away* from the crowd. Notice that? He then proceeded to speak to him using sign language, communicating in a way the man would understand. I love the visual of Jesus stepping into the man's quiet world.

In fact, as Jesus gets face-to-face with the sufferer, turn the volume all the way down in your mind until the silence is ringing in your head. Watch as Jesus puts his fingers into the man's ears. "See these?" Jesus motions and grins. "These are about to work." Then he touches the man's tongue. "Yes, son, this will work too." As Jesus looks up, I picture the man following Jesus' eyes and tilting his head back as well. And then it happened. Jesus sighed. My favorite part.

The sigh is a response to despair. Max Lucado says of the sigh, "In Heaven, you will be healthy. You never have been. Even on the days you felt fine, you weren't. You were a sitting duck for disease, infections, airborne bacteria, and microbes. This is a sigh of sadness, a deep breath, and a heavenly glance that resolves, 'It won't be this way for long.'"

It's true. On Earth, we have never been healthy. Jesus knew that. And his compassion and amazing pity came through that day for the deaf and mute the same way it showed up when Jesus cried outside the tomb of Lazarus. His heart breaks at the thought of ours stopping. We lose our memory, eyesight, and coordination. Cancer overtakes us and anxiety overwhelms us. Sleep eludes, fear consumes, and minds forget. The result of sin's presence by the fall of man rears its ugly head until we can't lift ours from the pillow. Such susceptibility took Christ's breath away.

Scientifically, a sigh is the brain's way of telling the lungs to refill themselves, and it comes at times of great sadness and emotion. When some people begged, pleaded, and implored of Christ on behalf of their needy friend, Jesus sighed as deeply as He cared. But rather than roar like Aslan, He tugged on ear lobes and touched a quiet tongue. *It won't be this way for long.*

> *On Earth, we have never been healthy.*

Oh, and I walked by the UPS Store recently. There's a new ramp and rails, and the doors will open automatically. Some people. I doubt they wore capes or had superhuman strength. They could have rolled in on skateboards wearing ball caps for all I know. But some people just came into town and said something.

~I Have to Go Back~

"His grief he will not forget; but it will not darken his heart, it will teach him wisdom."
— J.R.R. Tolkien

I wonder if I would have gone back. Ten lepers—lepers who were outcasts to society, unable to be with family and friends—saw Jesus and, from a safe distance, exercised faith. Let's read the powerful passage together.

"It happened that as he made his way toward Jerusalem, he crossed over the border between Samaria and Galilee. As he entered a village, ten men, all lepers, met him. They kept their distance but raised their voices, calling out, "Jesus, Master, have mercy on us!" Taking a good look at them, he said, "Go, show yourselves to the priests." They went, and while still on their way, became clean. One of them, when he realized that he was healed, turned around and came back, shouting his gratitude, glorifying God. He kneeled at Jesus' feet, so grateful. He couldn't thank him enough—and he was a Samaritan. Jesus said, "Were not ten healed? Where are the nine? Can none be found to come back and give glory to God except this outsider?" Then he said to him, "Get up. On your way. Your faith has healed and saved you." Luke 17: 11-19

First thing that jumps out of the story to me is the fact that they kept their distance. In that day and age, those suffering with leprosy weren't allowed near clean people, so they stuck to protocol behind an invisible, uncrossable border. Faces pressed against it, hands up, they did the only thing they could—scream. Their plea mirrored their pain. If octaves equaled misery, theirs was a high C. Then after a "good look at them," Jesus told them to go show the priests. Catch that? They figured they were keeping a safe distance, and yet Jesus got a *good* look at them. Wow. (I could get a full week of lessons from that one phrase.) And then, it happened. On their way to see the priests, new skin. Fingers replaced nubs. Faces filled voids. Thoughts of holding children and kissing spouses ran through their minds.

Now, one of them did what I hope I would do. He stopped.
Wait a second, he thought.

I cried,
He cared.
I moaned,
He gave mercy.
I have to go back.

And here's another great moment for me in this story. He came back shouting his praise. He figured if his suffering called for screaming, his healing called for hollering. But this time, no barrier. No outer marker. No holding pattern. He was clean and he knew it—and getting close to the One that made him that way was his default reaction. Like I said in the beginning, I wonder if I would have gone back. If not, may this little work be a step in His direction. Suffering sends you back.

~You Believed in Me~
"The Lord gets His best soldiers out of the highlands of affliction."
— Charles Spurgeon

Pastor Rick Warren enjoys telling a story that he had heard as a kid. You may have heard a version or two of it from *your* parents, but as the story goes, a group of 12 frogs were traveling together through a forest when two of them fell into a very deep, dark pit. The other 10 frogs gathered around the pit. When they realized how deep it was, they were certain that it was the end of their two friends.

The two frogs that had fallen into the pit started jumping with all their might in an attempt to get out. But from the perspective of safety, the other 10 frogs began to urge the trapped frogs to stop trying and just accept their fate. They kept yelling, "You're in too deep! There's no way you'll get out of this! It's impossible! Save your strength and die peacefully!"

But the two frogs at the bottom ignored the comments and kept trying to jump out, and still, the safe frogs kept yelling, "It's no use! It's hopeless! Save your energy!" Finally, one of the frogs in the pit got so discouraged by all the negativity that he gave up and died.

But the other frog at the bottom of the pit kept jumping harder and harder. And with every jump, he seemed to get stronger and stronger. It was an amazing effort to watch. Finally, he made it out to safety! The other frogs looked at him in astonishment and asked, "Why did you keep trying so hard when we were all urging you to give up?"

Interpreting what they said from their gestures, the frog explained, "Well, actually I'm deaf, so I couldn't hear a word you were saying. But I could see you were all shouting vigorously at me. I assumed it meant you believed I could make it and were encouraging me to not give up. So I was determined to keep trying as long as you believed in me!"

Powerful, huh? Not shocking, but I can't read that without crying. As a sentimental fool, I look at this story from so many angles. One that puts a lump in my throat is to consider the frog with special needs looking up

and seeing his buddies rooting for him. He wasn't gonna let them down.
Maybe he never felt like he had pals before; he never knew he was so
loved. Unlike his counterpart, he would die before he would quit. Yeah,
that gets me. I can relate to the frog that didn't quit.

***

Speaking of *pals,* the two lived on the same block as kids. Both had
strict, loving parents. Daily chores included loading hay, carrying feed,
and helping in the fields—and their young backs were growing strong
because of them. After school and homework, they'd meet up in the
street to play childhood games till dark. They were tight-knit. Best pals.

As it turned out, they had a mutual friend of the same age who lived
down the street. He couldn't walk; paralyzed from birth. But that didn't
stop him from telling a good joke or razzing the game's underdog. He
was part of the crew. One of the boys.

As the years passed, the boys grew into strong and able men with families of
their own. Except, of course, for the one who was crippled. His two buddies
checked on him daily though. He had a place at their tables on holidays.
He was the full-time ref in neighborhood competitions. They worshipped
together each weekend. Indeed, after all the years, they were still tight.

Well, when news arrived that *He* was in town, the two ran toward each
other's homes. In fact, they met in the middle and took turns catching
their breath as they talked about their plan. Strong boys became strong
men, and carrying their friend all the way across town to the One they
say was able to work miracles made all those childhood chores worth it.
In fact, those chores made it *possible.*

The crowd around their buddy's house made it tough to get inside
through traditional means. Holding the ends of the bed, the lifelong
friends looked at each other as if sharing the
same memory of hauling hay, hoisting feed,
playing games, and growing up. Only one
thing left for them to do: lift.
Most of us are familiar with
the *actual* Biblical account of the friends

> *I can relate to
> the frog that
> didn't quit.*

who lifted their friend through the roof to be healed… but isn't it neat to wonder what got them there? What we *do* know is that Jesus forgave sins, healed bones, and read minds.

Part of me likes to think that Jesus was pleased with the faith of those guys, a faith they exercised with their backs. And I like to imagine the three of them walking home together, don't you? Who knows, maybe they played a street game for old times' sake. Someone had some catching up to do.

~The Wedding Singer~

Take a saint and put him into any condition, and he knows how to rejoice in the Lord.
— Walter Cradock (1638)

Romania. Day one. Sitting in a makeshift waiting room, I'm reminded of the blind man sitting on the side of the road in Jericho. His name was Bartimaeus, and when he heard it was Jesus walking by, he began to shout out, "Jesus, Son of David, have mercy on me!" Over and over he yelled. Despite being rebuked by others, he continued to shout, "Jesus, Son of David, have mercy on me!" And it's the reaction of Jesus that captures me in this moment. The Bible says that when Jesus heard him shouting, He "stopped walking." Some Bible versions say that He "stood still," and other translations say He "stopped in His tracks." I'll come back to that.

With a fancy camera I'm still learning to use, I crouch in the corner among the families awaiting wheelchairs and Bibles. As an old writer, the assignment on this Wheels for the World outreach felt natural enough— *easy.* Capture the scene. Document the story. What I didn't expect was the scene or the story.

From what I could tell, nobody dropped him off. Nobody escorted him in. He made his way to us on his hands. Using two wooden blocks about the size of bricks, adorned with homemade handles—picture two Olympic pommel horse grips—Florin (pronounced *Floor-een*), 41, made his way inside the venue to wait his turn. With his legs coiled up underneath him, this is how he's been entering rooms since he was 5 years old.

With the blocks of wood now serving as his seat in the holding area, you could tell he was no stranger to tight quarters. As our eyes met, I smiled gently. He didn't. The look on *his* face said that he had seen the look on *my* face many times before. I'm pretty sure I turned away first. Gulp. With tears already streaming down my face and onto my camera, I found myself longing for his name to be called, for him to get his first wheelchair, and for him to hear that Jesus loves him; just hurry with all of it, please.

As we waited, I wondered what kind of adversity he'd endured over the course of his life. Something tells me he's been sitting on the side of that dusty road in Jericho.

Well, although he was a bit camera shy at first, by the time he made his way into the distribution center, he had become fast friends with the entire room—including, if I'm not mistaken, a marriage proposal to one of Joni's most faithful volunteers, Susan, who was serving on something like her 20th Wheels trip.

Florin's face was dark, with thick leathery skin and pronounced grooves in his cheeks that deepened as he smiled. His raspy voice was a testament to, and likely a byproduct of, one of his many talents and means of income—part-time wedding singer. With a lump in my throat, I emerged from behind the safety of my camera and extended my hand to shake his. His rough palm was jet black. His big strong fingers swallowed mine. I squeezed harder as if to initiate a grip challenge, and he returned the favor with a confident grin. (He won.)

As the experts on the team worked on a chair that would be ideal for Florin, we learned that his legs stopped working at the age of 5. After a failed surgery 20 years ago, along with no medical care since, he's done his best with the least. He lives with his brother and finds work in the fields. His chair almost complete, we gave him Joni Eareckson Tada's book and began laying the groundwork for the Gospel message that would soon be delivered to him by the in-country pastors.

Long story short, when his wheelchair was presented, we had to hold him back. Once we explained the details and the ins and outs of the chair, he was simply done listening. He transferred himself into the chair with reckless abandon and began to sing. His powerful hands maneuvered the wheelchair around the room with childlike faith and a refreshing, natural fearlessness that seemed to rub off on all of us.

By the time a new set of families had entered the building, Florin was outside in his new wheelchair. On his lap sat a pair of worn-out wooden blocks and a Bible. I was told that Florin hadn't heard about the wheelchair outreach in Romania until the night before. My gut tells me he didn't want the Lord to take another sweet step, so he stole that line from Bartimaeus and got up.

Speaking of which, when Bartimaeus received his sight, the Bible says that the very first thing he did was follow Jesus along the road. I suppose he figured the best way to test his new eyes was to focus on the One who finally made them work.

I like to think that Florin is doing the very same thing.

~Go and Do the Work~

My joy in life does not come from being physically fit. And God's love is not dependant on my ability to walk.
— Barry Funnell

D iving deep into the subject of weakness and suffering, and how God uses such, I've learned that the likes of the Apostle Paul and Job and Jacob and Moses all had disabilities or chronic illnesses to reveal God's power and to help them realize their smallness and dependence. Barry was no different.

With dreams of becoming a rich dentist, traveling the world on holidays and playing golf on Wednesdays, Barry Funnell, who loved bodybuilding and being the class clown was in his second year of school when all of that changed. He and a buddy wanted to impress some girls, so they decided to climb onto the roof of a gymnasium which was adjacent to the female dormitory. Unable to find an opening, they decided to turn back. That's when Barry's foot slipped through a skylight.

Hours later Barry woke up in the hospital with his spinal cord completely severed. Unable to feel his legs, his thoughts raced back to his days as a boy when he gave his life to Christ, was baptized by his dad and then how he ran away from God to pursue all sorts of other pleasures. He was haunted by the thought that he had never shared the love of Jesus with anyone. He had been "too cool" for that, he realized. He laid in the hospital for weeks and months reading his Bible, recommitting his life to Christ and leaning on God for encouragement.

"Lying paralyzed in my hospital bed, I recommitted my life fully to God. I repented of my wrongdoings, my pride. I asked God to forgive me and to pick up the broken pieces of my life and use me as he saw fit. I felt embarrassed that I had so often endangered myself due to seeking an adrenaline rush and wanting to impress others instead of living my life for him. My spinal cord completely severed, I had to face the prospect of spending the rest of my life in a wheelchair. A major part of my rehab was gaining the ability to empty my bladder via self-catheterization and also to evacuate my bowel manually. I can say this was, and still is, the most difficult and awkward aspect of paraplegia." - Disability in Mission:

The Church's Hidden Treasure" by David Deuel.

At the time that this chapter was being written, my wife was studying and preparing to lead a Bible study for hundreds of women in our local community. They were studying the Book of James. Known as the Proverbs of the New Testament, James puts faith to work. It's the *show me* book. If you love me, show me.

> *Words, words, words!*
> *Sing me no song.*
> *Read me no rhyme.*
> *Don't waste my time, Show me.*
> *Don't talk of June,*
> *Don't talk of fall.*
> *Don't talk at all. Show me.*

That's not from the Book of James, of course, but those are the piercing lyrics from *My Fair Lady*. I can empathize with Audrey Hepburn being "up to here" with words. *My own*, that is. That's why the story of Barry is so uplifting.

While in his fourth year of dental studies Barry met his future wife Julia. They became medical missionaries but grew a passion for Bible translation. "People do need good health and strong teeth, but we sensed our passion was to instead give them a lasting gift; the Word of God which will never pass away."

Along with their three adopted children, they have checked over fifty different Bible translations for accuracy and travel to South East Asia and Africa ten times a year. He relies on God to help him in every situation in developing countries. From waiting on buses or in getting help on airplanes, his dependence on God in the mundane only grows his faith. He once hand-cycled 1600km to raise money for Bible translation. It took him 23 days.

"My joy in life does not come from being physically fit," he says. "And God's love is not dependent on my ability to walk. My disability has taught me how insignificant working legs are in the light of souls and their eternal wellbeing."

Guys, this is "faith & fitness." You can't fit it on a shirt, drink it in a supplement, or grasp it in a CrossFit workout. "Faith & fitness" is just a made up phrase - just words - without real, inner work that glorifies God and serves others; the only kind of work that will last. I see the realness in people like Barry Funnell. Thrust into God's work and sent to the mission field as a paraplegic, the former bodybuilder doesn't let his body distract him from honoring God with it.

He travels the world and translates the Bible, and all he needs is a little help with stairs. And in case you were wondering, Barry stays active to keep fit for the mission field. He swims twice a week and took up sailing. And yes, he plays golf once a week; usually on Wednesdays.

> *Guys, this is "faith & fitness." You can't fit it on a shirt, drink it in a supplement, or grasp it in a CrossFit workout.*

REFLECTION

Then I heard the voice of the Lord saying, "Whom shall I send? And who will go for us?"
And I said, "Here am I. Send me!"(Isaiah 6:8)

You know the scene. You've planned your workout with pristine precision. You've prepped yourself with enough fast-digesting protein and slow-digesting carbs to pull a train across town. But as you try to leave the house, you can't find your keys. Once you do, you realize you have about enough gasoline to get that train 10 feet. Ugh. Ok. Gasoline? Check. So, you made it to the gym, but based on the lack of parking, you figure the entire side of town decided to train this day. *Really?*

Ok. You're in. But dang. The guy at the front desk is moving at a glacial pace scanning membership cards! Doesn't he know how important your workout is and how precious your time is to do it? Good grief. *Finally!!* You're in. The promised land. Your *little kingdom*. **Your world**. You find your locker, use the restroom. You're ready. Then you make your way to the machine you've been dying to use only to find that the person on it seems to have put up a mailbox, a welcome mat and a bird feeder. He is not leaving anytime soon. Argh!!

Sound far-fetched? Well, if I'm not describing you, I'm probably describing me in my old gym days. (Boy, don't we miss the meaning?) For all we know, the delay in finding your keys and the empty gas tank allowed an emergency vehicle a clear path to their destination. The full parking lot wasn't a bunch of newcomers, they were visitors from a local mission shelter that needed to use the showers and facilities. And the guy working the front desk, he's impacted by special abilities. He's worked his way through school to earn his high school diploma. The gym owner gave him a chance to work a few hours each day. This is his first week on the register. He gets nervous when he's alone and he doesn't remember how to print the receipt.

And oh, the guy on the machine? You know, the one that seems to have taken up residence? Well, he's just a guy; someone's son and brother. He's battled addiction and he lost his mother to cancer. He's single, and he's given up hope of ever finding someone to love. He doesn't know how to work this machine, let alone what muscles it works. He's just a sweet guy with a soft heart. He shows up at the gym just to be around people and to take care of his health as best he can. He figures the crowded parking lot means the odds are good that he may meet a friend or two. Someone who may smile his way. Someone to say hello. Someone to show him how to train on this complicated machine. Someone to give love a face.

When grace walks in the gym, pride slips out the back.

When "faith & fitness" meets grace in suffering, directions change, hearts break.

"How many more sets you got?" you ask.

I write that scenario to help illustrate an important point. Training or fitness can be an expression of worship or praise, of course, but it falls short. Why? Only until we serve others by it and because of it can we truly be fulfilled. Only serving God and others truly completes the effort. Feeling strong and looking great will not be enough. You have to do something that will outlast your atrophy to find fulfillment.

Adam and Eve were the first to suffer body image issues. When they lost perfection, shame and insecurities set it. Since then, it's been a fight. Fitness people will tell you, "It's about progress, not perfection." When actually, it is ALL about perfection; not in our ability to achieve it, but in our loss of it. And our broken lives and groaning bodies are the result of a fallen, sinful nature. Simple as that.

Serving others completes the purpose of the gift of health. In some ways, it's very similar to what C.S. Lewis said about praise. "I think we delight to praise what we enjoy because the praise not merely expresses but completes the enjoyment; it is its appointed consummation."

Training in and of itself isn't enough. From experience, the byproducts of effort won't suffice. At the end of the day, the grit, the progress, the change, the pump and the reflection will be accompanied by an emptiness. We may not perceive it or even be able to put our finger on it, but we think it's just a drive we have inside us that can be satisfied by hitting it again the next day and "crushing" goals or pushing ourselves to the limit. But the cycle of the fight is a mindless, meaningless loop unless we serve someone in need. The atrophy that occurs overnight needs more than another regimen, it needs a reason.

***

God created the Heavens and the earth, along with your neighborhood, and the mountains, and your little gym, and billions of galaxies, each grain of sand on every seashore, the hummingbird's wings, and the brittle bones of the hands typing this poorly constructed sentence for one purpose: for the glory of God's grace. That's it. Why does He allow for both fitness and suffering? Why does He approve health *and* illness? To display the glory of His grace.

John Piper says, "God created man in his own image. What was the point? The point of an image is to point to the original. Glorify the original. God made humans in his image so that the world would be filled with reflectors of God."

Your best health will come when your body points others to Christ. That may not mean your idea of an "ideal" weight. That may not come after your best lift, run, or set. It may even come on your weakest, toughest, sickest day. But the best moment your body will ever experience is when the glory of His grace is on display. Your best moment of bodily stewardship won't come at the end of a grueling set and with a pump to promote, but in how you treat others along the way and serving their needs.

In his book *Walking with God Through Pain and Suffering*, Tim Keller reveals countless concepts of the origins of suffering, its purpose, the byproducts, and more, but there are a few major points I will list here, as they are critical for our industry.

» *Suffering has the potential of giving us a more accurate appraisal of our own limitations.*

» *Suffering also leads us to examine ourselves and see weaknesses, because it brings out the worst in us. Our weak faith, sharp tongues, laziness, insensitivity to people, worry, bitter spirit, and other weaknesses in character become evident to us and others in hard times.*

» *Suffering changes the relationship to the good things in our lives. We will see that some things have become too important to us. It fortifies us against being too cast down by future reversals. It also brings us new sources of joy we were not tapping before.*

I remember sitting in the office of the former president of a very prominent charity. We had a great chat. He asked me about my life and career and after I had listed all the things I'd done, he said something that rocked me. He said, "Jimmy, you've had a lot of success, but what would your life look like if things really turned out well?" Talk about blow to the ego. I had just listed my accomplishments but he was looking for substance. His ears were conditioned to notice significance rather than success.

Fortunately for me these days, suffering and pain, the re-arranging of my priorities and the exposure to those impacted by special needs have helped me realize what is significant and what is not. You can take all the books and success and the silly kingdoms of goals away, because the joy of the gift of health will atrophy, decay and die if not expressed in the service to those in need. If we waste in on self, it will do just that. We have to serve. Our hard work won't be satisfied without it.

> *The gift of health will atrophy, decay and die if not expressed in the service to those in need. If we waste in on self, it will do just that. We have to serve. Our hard work won't be satisfied without it.*

CROSSING JORDAN

I couldn't take my eyes off of Bodexpress. As soon as the race began, I called downstairs for Loretta because she *needed* to come watch this with me. "Hurry! There's a horse running without a jockey at the Preakness," I said with elevating octaves of joy. The jockey had fallen off the horse (unharmed) and I literally stood in my living room with a lump in my throat as I clapped with sincere hope. Such a sweet moment. Tears were inevitable.

While War of Will won the Preakness, Bodexpress won my heart and the hearts of millions. I fell back into my chair as exhausted as I was exhilarated. Deep sigh of happiness. It had been a long time since I'd watched a scene so awesome. He just wanted to run with his friends. He was like, "Hey guys, wait for me!" In fact, I remember noticing him being jumpy and jittery at the gate. He was trapped for a minute. But then...*freedom.*

The next day, out of the blue, Gina Spivey, the Pastor of the special needs ministry at our church, sent me a picture of my boy Jordan. He was—wait for it—standing next to a horse. Yep. The timing was surreal. Not sure of the context of the pic; not sure if he rode the horse that day (he's been riding horses since he was 3) or if Jordan was merely there to walk him and care for him. I love him so much. In some ways, Jordan is trapped inside. Autism saddles his mind and reins his thoughts. He's got the sweetest heart of any boy you've ever met, and every so often, it'll happen.

Jordan will look me *square* in the eye, and he'll say something or respond to something with absolute coherence and lucidity. As if waking up from a dream, he'll look at me inquisitively, almost as if he's wondering how long I'd been sitting there. I can't explain it, but he locks on to the topic. And when he does, I can't take my eyes off of him. I delicately respond with a follow-up and try to keep him on track before we change universes. But for just a split second, we have a typical conversation. As if for the briefest of moments, he's free.

Sometimes moments of purity invite themselves into our world without notice, permission, or apology. Those moments don't always last.

Speaking of, Bodexpress decided to run around the track one more time after the race, just for the fun of it. The handlers eventually caught up with him and escorted him back to his stall, but one more time around the track was just too irresistible.

(Nine years earlier)

"You like mustard?"

"Yes. I like mustard," I replied.

Optimistic but being thorough, Jordan leaned his little head to the side. "What color is mustard?"

"Yellow. Mustard is yellow," I said with certainty.

Pause.

"Whaaaat's yellow?" (As if he was giving me sort of a final exam; maybe to see if I was—and would always be—*paying attention*.)

"Mustard," I testified (and with an assurance that I always would be listening).

Then he reached for my hand. I like to think that meant he thought I was alright. Then we walked to put his lunch pail away and that was that. That was the day I met Jordan. We've been best pals ever since. When we first started hanging out, he'd refer to me as *the little guy that helps him*. How spot-on was he about that?

Don't tell Gina, but Jordan and I used to take the toys out of the toy room, slam the outside gate, and sometimes we threw things over the fence. And every now and again, when he was smiling, jumping, and giggling to himself, I imagined that he'd just heard something that only he and God could hear, and I got to watch him run.

You know, after countless Buddy Breaks and Respite opportunities, a thousand fish tacos in Malibu, and more post-church French toast than my 50-year-old body is allowed, I have no doubt I'm closer to Jesus when I'm with Jordan. Not because of anything in me, but because if anything in life is pure and good and right and excellent, it's found in the hearts and minds of kids with special needs. It's like I'm closer to Heaven itself. Jordan and his friends take me higher. Without trying, they teach me what it means to be kind, forgiving, fun, and innocent. And when I come down again, I'm different. Sweeter. Gentler. And in some ways, tougher.

***

Big Bear, California. The small town 100 miles east of Los Angeles is hallowed training ground. Resting 9,000 feet above sea level and surrounded by the San Bernardino National Forest, Big Bear Lake is seven miles long and about a half-mile wide. With more than 300 days of sunshine each year, the haven is above the pollution, above the clouds, above the noise. And for many a boxer, the rare air is fertile terrain for the most rigorous and guided of training schemes.

Years ago I spent time training in an altitude chamber. As you may know, training at altitude helps you perform better at sea level. The more time you spend up high, the better you perform down low. As an old exercise physiologist, that makes good sense to me, but the way Jordan and his friends impact my heart makes it true. Spend time on high and you will perform better on the ground.

I think that's why, after I leave his presence or I say goodbye to all of the kids after a day of respite, the places we go and the crowds we encounter later in the day get the best version of me. I'm more patient in line at the supermarket or more forgiving on the road. I smile more and demonstrate more compassion at the mall or in restaurants. Why? Because joy doesn't wear off that fast. You don't get over it quickly. It takes time for my natural inclinations to return. I don't know. I just fight a better fight when I'm full of the good stuff of life. The kind of traits or fruits of the Spirit that God wants me to demonstrate are the ones I'm taught by those impacted by disabilities. That's not an exaggeration.

Aaron Cohen once wrote, *Boxers are products of place; inevitably where they come from is how they end up in the ring, and how they fight once they get there.* Genius. And true. Not just for boxers. And not just for washed-up writers. There's not a person on Earth tougher than a parent of a child impacted by special needs. There's more heart and nerve and life and torment and joy and heartache and love in one breath of a mother caring for her disabled child than those that come from a thousand rounds inside the ring.

As I was writing this manuscript, Jordan's mom, Mendy, delivered a body blow—one that buckled both me and Loretta.

"I don't know how to say this," she texted to Loretta after weeks of dread. "I can't bring myself to tell Jimmy, but we are moving away to be closer to family and better schools for Jordan."

When we met up in person a couple days later to talk about it, I remember her explaining, "Tennessee isn't that far. We know so many people there, and don't worry, we will Facetime and visit often, and we will see each other on holidays..." As if her voice was fading into the background, all I could picture was Jordan leaving.

My buddy for nearly a decade was about to pack up and drive out of town. Now, that may not seem like a ton of bricks to you, but I assure you the news was too heavy for these narrow shoulders. Loretta and I held each other tight that night and just cried at the news. What would we do without him?

Because Jordan brings so much meaning to our world, it took a while to accept and process this news. In fact, I think we are *still* doing those things. That's not hyperbole. His presence in our lives helps balance the stresses of work and personal health battles and chronic pain. He motivates me at work, and he unknowingly helps me manage the unusual stresses of my life in hospitality. He's someone we just love to hang with, and someone we simply need in our day-to-day lives.
But let me try to put something into words. When we are with the kids

who are affected by disabilities, we're of course there to have a blast and make sure they are safe, but one of our primary purposes is to **allow the** parents and caregivers a much-needed rest—what we call respite. You've heard me discuss how important that is, but Loretta and I will tell you that *we* are the beneficiaries. We're the ones being blessed. We're the ones resting.

I enjoy explaining this to Gina because it's like describing to Derek Jeter what it's like to field a ground ball. She gets it. When I'm with Jordan and his friends for a time of respite care, I'm the one getting the rest. It's like I've been outside all day long and it's my turn at the water fountain. Refreshment of my soul. And when it's over and the parents have collected their kiddos, we're exhausted and completely and utterly filled. We can't take any more goodness.

Imagine driving your car non-stop across the country. No sleep, few bathroom stops, fast food, laughter, tears, amazing stories, and a million different topics of discussion—but eventually you arrive at your destination. Your car is overheated and needs a serious wash, new tires, an oil change, and has a few thousand more miles on it. But when you look at your tank, it reads *full*. That's what it's like after respite.

You would love Jordan. He's never met a stranger. Says hello to all *the ladies*. Even the girls he's already spoken to earlier in the day, he makes sure they know he's around. And Jordan absorbs his surroundings and the feelings his friends are experiencing.

One day, Jordan and I were playing board games when one of his buddies, Johnny, began to have a bit of a tough time. Johnny is non-verbal and highly emotional at times. At the time, the special abilities area was in the midst of a facelift and we had to retreat into unfamiliar areas of the church. The change was a little more than Johnny could bear. So he broke down. And when he cried, Jordan noticed and began to do what Jordan does: he looked on the bright side. "Johnny's just having a tough time. He's sad that we're in this room. Johnny will be okay." All of which I agreed with.

But as we continued to play our game, I noticed that Jordan was continuously looking back at Johnny. At this point, Johnny was going in and out of his own pain. Minutes of dry eyes were followed by minutes of tears. This went on for some time. And Jordan, who typically keeps a stiff upper lip, began to feel for Johnny. Tears filled his eyes, the corners of his mouth began to droop, and he started to cry—so much so that he continued to share in Johnny's travail like I'd never seen before.

Jordan kept saying, "Johnny is so sad. He's just so sad about this room. But Johnny is gonna be alright." Hours went by. Every few minutes, the thought of Johnny having a tough time was enough to bring Jordan's emotions to multiple breaking points. I'd watch as he wiped his face of the tears. Even when Johnny wasn't in the room, Jordan was feeling for his friend. Guys, he's the kindest, sweetest young man you'd ever want to meet.

By the time respite was over, I think everyone was exhausted. Johnny and Jordan were both dry-eyed and playing with their friends and ready to see Mom and Dad. I was a wreck. But the experience remains with me to this very day. I am at my best when I'm with him and his friends in church. Why? Because they live how we should live; they react as we should react. They rejoice with others and they weep with those that weep. Name a fruit of the spirit and you'll find it in someone at respite.

As I mentioned, Jordan has since moved away. He's making friends, adjusting to his new room at home, and he's taking the special needs bus to school all by himself. I know that as he steps onto the playground and into his classroom, he's asking all the right questions, saying hello to every girl, remaining positive, and just being himself. He's my best pal. And much like he did with me in sharing memories from the time before we met, I like to think that someone he's talking to is hearing about his adventures with Jimmy.

Do you know my friend Jimmy? Yeah. He's the little guy that helps me.

Behind The 2: MOBILITY & RESPITE

What was the first thing you did when you woke up this morning? It's likely you had to move.

Try to imagine life without mobility. We've seen it. We've traveled the neighborhoods, we've found the alleys, and we've been in the lonely rooms. We've seen people like Floreen in Romania, who I met on a Wheels for the World trip, walking on his hands and wearing his Sunday best, because the day you get a wheelchair is the most important day of your life.

Seventy million people live without the gift of mobility. Shamed, and in some cases, forgotten or abandoned. Trapped, as if in a cellar with no stairs or a prison with no key. Mobility would change everything. They just need wheelchairs. In this world, some people can't move.

And others, well, others can't stop. Parents, grandparents, and caregivers of those with special needs operate in a world of perpetual motion, propelled by the affection of those they hold closest. And while life is full of endless joys, research shows that the emotional and physical stress can be overwhelming. They need rest. They need respite.

Respite can come in many forms, like getting fresh air at the market, having a date with a spouse, or a nap with a side of Netflix.

But imagine not having the luxury of a full night's sleep or time for a walk. It can be an existence of deficit, fatigue, and stress—the kind that stalls hope and drains the soul.

In the end, few scenes produce images as startling as disability among the poor or the exhaustion of a guardian. They provide indisputable evidence of just how much life demands of the will.

Fitness—regardless of the sport or activity—is very much a meld of mobility and respite. Whether you lift weights or ride bikes, training is, in its purest sense, a cascading sequence of miracles—work followed by rest, a chain of events known to a rare breed as gifts of grace. Joni

Eareckson Tada once said, "The hallmark of a healthy society has always been measured by how it cares for the disadvantaged."

Even though fitness is often measured by what is visible, the impact is eternally based in what is not. Mobility and Respite. 2 Causes, One Body. Some people can't move. Others can't stop.

This little book was written to help.

Notes and References

PREFACE:
Be Gone, Unbelief, Olney Hymns

INTRODUCTION:
The Chronicles of Narnia, C.S. Lewis
The Road to Character by David Brooks

SECTION 1:
The Beyond Suffering Bible, Joni Eareckson Tada
The Pursuit of God, A.W. Tozer
Job's Resignation, The Spurgeon Center, C. H. Spurgeon
Walking with God through Pain and Suffering, Tim Keller
Broken Praise, Todd Smith, Music Inspire by The Story
Hymns of Suffering, Crossway Books, Joni Eareckson Tada
He Still Moves Stones, Max Lucado
Suffering, Gospel Hope When Nothing Makes Sense, Paul Tripp
Seasons of Sorrow, Tim Challies

SECTION TWO:
Christian George, The Spurgeon Center
I am not, but I know I Am, Louie Giglio
The Road to Character, David Brooks
Truth for Life, Alistair Begg
Suffering, Gospel Hope When Nothing Makes Sense, Paul Tripp

SECTION THREE:
Disability in Mission, The Church's Hidden Treasure, David Deuel,
Joni & Friends International Disability Center
Show Me, My Fair Lady
Walking with God Through Pain and Suffering, Tim Keller

www.ingramcontent.com/pod-product-compliance
Lightning Source LLC
Chambersburg PA
CBHW031542260326
41914CB00002B/226